MASTER RECIPES FROM
THE HERBAL APOTHECARY

# Master Recipes

## FROM THE Herbal Apothecary

**375** TINCTURES, SALVES, TEAS, CAPSULES, OILS AND WASHES FOR **WHOLE BODY HEALTH** AND **WELLNESS**

## JJ PURSELL

WITH PHOTOS BY SHAWN LINEHAN

Timber Press

Portland, Oregon

This book is dedicated to Tommy, my sweet, funny, lovable boy.

Copyright © 2019 by JJ Pursell. All rights reserved.

Photo and illustration credits appear on page 279.

Published in 2019 by Timber Press, Inc.

The Haseltine Building
133 S.W. Second Avenue, Suite 450
Portland, Oregon 97204-3527
timberpress.com

Printed in China

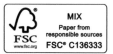

Text and cover design by Hillary Caudle

ISBN 978-1-60469-852-7

Catalog records for this book are available from the Library of Congress and the British Library.

# CONTENTS

# INTRODUCTION

WELCOME! If you've found yourself here, it's likely because you want to feel empowered to care for yourself and your family with herbs as an alternative to over-the-counter or prescription pharmaceuticals for common ailments. Or maybe you are seeking knowledge about the traditional ways of healing for an ongoing health issue. Perhaps you've already begun exploring herbal medicine and have developed a more serious interest—you are ready to learn and to incorporate herbal remedies into your daily self-care routine. Whatever the reason, I invite you to explore the recipes that follow at your own pace and as you need them.

When I was a budding herbal enthusiast in my twenties, I referred to books very similar to this one but often had to look in multiple volumes to find what I needed. In this book, I've done my best to create an inclusive, concise reference that is easy to use. The first chapter provides you with basic recipes for the thirteen most useful delivery methods and applications of herbal remedies—along with background about which is best suited to what type of ailment and why. It also describes sixty herbs that are basics in the medicine cabinet. The following thematic chapters provide treatments for ailments from A to Z. Everything you need in order to incorporate herbs into your daily life with the goal of achieving balanced overall health and improved wellness is here.

More and more, we are returning to the ways of self-reliance and traditional medicine. Herbal medicine is an important tool for helping us live healthier lives and actively participating in improving our overall health, naturally. You might use herbs as part of a daily routine or step it up when something acute shows up at your door. Studying the plants—their ethnobotanical and folk uses and the science of the chemical composition that makes them powerful healing agents—gives herbalists and naturopathic physicians like me a framework for prescribing and creating treatments.

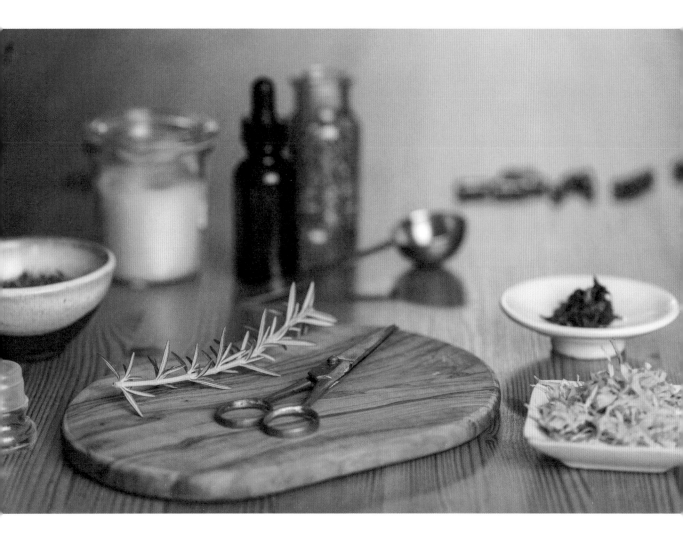

In writing this book, I reflected on my patients' and customers' most common requests and then created 375 recipes to address these concerns. The recipes will teach you how to manage day-to-day physical complaints such as colds, headaches, stomach upset, and stress. One powerful reason for turning to herbal medicine is that it provides access to healing medicine on the spot, hours or days before you could even get a doctor's appointment. If you sprain your ankle playing basketball, for example, and you know that witch hazel leaf and bark can reduce swelling and pain, you can immediately apply a poultice to get ahead of the inflammation process. Another example is having catnip and fennel seed tea on hand to provide instant relief from overindulging at dinner or for general stomach upset.

You may already take herbs, vitamins, and supplements regularly. That market has exploded during the last quarter of a century, encouraging us to take this or that capsule or tablet to regain health and attain vital longevity. The upside to this is that as a result, much scientific research and education has been dedicated to natural health products. This has provided consumers with real information regarding what they are taking and what is realistic as far as expected results.

We are lucky to live in a time when medical science and advanced treatments are available to us. I am personally thankful for Western medicine and hospitals, as I have benefited greatly from modern medicine and feel truly blessed to live in a place where we have relatively easy access to it. I mention this because even though I am dedicated to natural medical practices as a naturopathic physician, licensed acupuncturist, and herbalist, I believe there is a time and place for all types of medical practice. As with most things, finding balance is necessary. What appeals to me about herbal medicine is its accessibility, and one of the reasons I became a naturopathic physician is my belief in empowering others to care for themselves, naturally, whenever possible. I don't believe there should be as large a gap between people and their health care as currently exists in most Western countries.

In my view, all doctors should be teachers, helping their patients learn about their bodies and the ways in which they heal. Too often we're simply shepherded through an impersonal health care system and given a quick fix without an education about how to avoid the same problem in the future or any information on how what we're taking affects our body's natural systems. If you arm yourself with the knowledge in this volume, you'll be able to reclaim sovereignty over your own health and you will feel confident about treating yourself for any of the dozens of common issues listed here. When we do this, we form a relationship with our body. As our awareness grows of how our body feels when it's in balance, we gain keen insight into its form and function, and we're better able to identify any imbalances.

How and why herbs work is something of an esoteric conversation. I could provide endless citations of scientific papers on the effects of specific plant constituents, but the total healing effect of an herb on the body is more than the sum of its parts. Let's take echinacea as an example. Echinacea is one of the most researched herbs, with most researchers isolating individual components of the root to identify the actions it produces in the body. This is the most common way for researchers to study an herb, by taking it apart and looking at each part individually. The most prominent parts (constituents) of

*Echinacea purpurea* are caffeic acid derivatives (phenolic compounds), alkamides, and polysaccharides. Research shows that caffeic acid derivatives are potent antioxidants that have important anti-inflammatory effects. Alkamides have stimulatory effects on phagocytosis (they destroy foreign cell types) and trigger effects on the pro-inflammatory cytokines. Cytokines are cell-signaling molecules that aid cell-to-cell communication in immune responses and stimulate the movement of cells toward sites of inflammation, infection, and trauma.

My point here is that research is a great way to identify the individual components of an herb and their actions. This serves an educational purpose and adds to the body of scientific knowledge about plants looked to by those who prefer to rely on science as they consider how to incorporate herbs into their lives. But, and I'm guessing you were feeling the *but* coming, the scientific research method misses a key point: herbs and the greater plant kingdom in general don't work because or when their specific components are isolated. Each plant has an evolved series of complex systems that work symbiotically when all parts function together. And our bodies have evolved right along with them.

It's possible, for example, for one herb to contain elements that individually have contradictory actions such as moistening and drying or astringing and dilating. It seems odd, perhaps, until you think that herbs must be self-sufficient to survive in the wild. They must have many different mechanisms in order to handle various conditions, and they turn to different parts of their own natures as needed to respond to them. Therein lies the magic and wisdom of nature. Plants have adapted to become resilient, which in turn reduces the organism's potential for stress. Yes, stress. Like us, a plant that isn't getting what it needs will produce a stress response—and we all know the impact stress has on our health. Since they can't take themselves to the doctor, plants evolved defense mechanisms.

One of the most frequent questions I hear from people beginning an herbal medicine regimen is: How does an herb know where it's needed in the body? Using our echinacea example again, someone might ask: How does it know to go to my nose and head to relieve cold symptoms? Well, an herb responds in much the same way as a pain reliever like Tylenol. Both are responding to messages the brain receives from the body. When you experience pain or symptoms in your body, certain chemicals are released. These chemicals contain messages and these messages are sent to the brain to alert it of what and where the issue is. When you take medicine, its goal is to find where the messages are coming from so it can help. Once it does, it turns off the chemical response, calms the reaction, and returns the physiological function back to normal. It also offers healing constituents to do its best to correct the problem. This is where the multitude

9

of varying actions really shines. Whereas a drug often has one action, an herb can offer many different supporting actions. And if you blend herbs together—for example, echinacea and myrrh, traditionally used to treat pain and inflammation—you begin to create a dynamic medicinal force that can directly soothe your symptoms.

So what balance do you personally want to strike between letting science and experience guide your personal herbal journey? Perhaps you want to get deep into herbs' biological constituents, learning classifications and their actions, in which case I'd refer you to my previous volume, *The Herbal Apothecary*. Or maybe you'd rather learn experientially, taking in a recommended plant as a tea or tincture and recording your personal experience with it. The more you use herbs, the more they will become like trusted friends you can call upon whenever you need them. Personally, I have a biochemistry past and have spent many years looking into plants' scientific natures, so thinking about the positive chemical interactions they can create reinforces my personal experience of what folk and ethnic practitioners have long trusted. As with any passion that lasts a lifetime, the body of knowledge you'll accumulate through your own practice will become a part of you, part of your daily life.

Herbs take center stage for the majority of the recipes in this book, but I have also added occasional suggestions from naturopathic and traditional Chinese medicine—sometimes an old nature cure recipe just can't be beat. Each recipe is described by application (tea, tincture, capsule, poultice, oil, and so on) and then use (cough, ache, and so forth). As you get more comfortable with your herbal use and studies, you can begin to interchange application types—meaning you can turn a tea recipe into a tincture recipe, or a tincture recipe into a capsule recipe.

The bulk of the book begins with recipes focused on day-to-day complaints and how to treat them. This includes such things as acne, gas, and insomnia. The next section is dedicated to immune health and ways to support the body through the season of colds and flus. Separate sections for women and men highlight general, common health issues. The next section is for our children, providing safe and simple ways to help them move through troubles such as fever, earaches, and tummy aches. Then there is a section on herbal medicine for emotional balance. Having herbs on hand when you are traveling can be a lifesaver, so I've also included a group of recipes to help you prepare an herbal traveling kit. The next section is dedicated to my mom and the elders of our community. These recipes are specific to the complaints that tend to come along as we age even if we are vibrant in spirit and young at heart. Last I've included an odds-and-ends section to address animal care, natural dyeing, and homekeeping with unique applications of herbs from years gone by.

The goal of this book is to provide safe and effective herbal recipes that anyone can use. My wish for the book is that it is relevant and helpful. I've created a layout that makes it easy to find specific recipes right when you need them. At times different conditions require different preparations—for example, for the body surface, sometimes a salve is indicated, other times a poultice, and yet other times a wash. This is the beauty of having choices. It allows you to treat effectively with the best course of action. While there are hundreds of herbs that could possibly be used, the herbs used in these recipes are considered universally safe for general consumption and are readily available at your local herb shop (shop local!) or, if needed, online (fettlebotanic.com).

As with any self-care practice, it's important to understand when you need to seek professional help. The recipes in this book are meant to be used for personal health and well-being. They are not meant to cure debilitating illness or serious conditions. While the herbs mentioned in this book are all considered generally safe by the FDA, I believe it is always best to consult your practitioner before taking herbs internally to ensure safety and to support your knowledge of herbal medicine.

My hope is that over the years your copy of this book will become well worn from use, dog-eared and marked up with personal notes throughout. May these recipes bring you relief, vitality, and the comfort of knowing you can care for yourself. May we all benefit from the gift of healing plants.

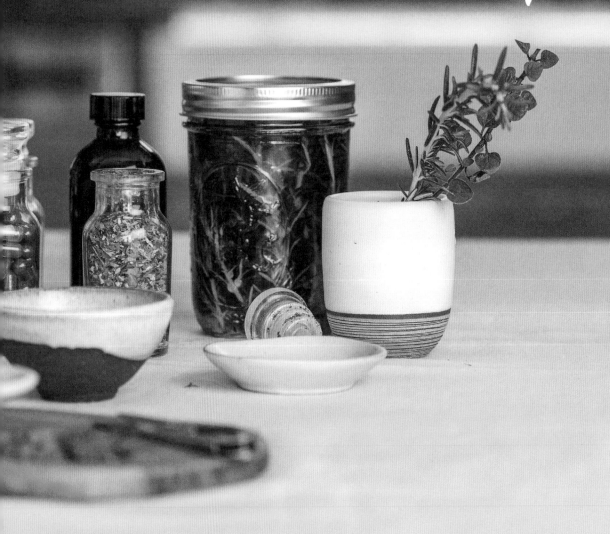

# Master Recipes

THE FIRST STEP IN LEARNING how to use herbs effectively as medicine is educating yourself about the various ways they can be applied or ingested. This chapter details the most common ways to use herbs. As I mentioned earlier, different preparations are recommended for different conditions. If I need headache relief quickly, I tend to choose a tincture, whereas if my stomach is upset I typically drink a cup of soothing tea. First I'll discuss various types of herbal products—teas, tinctures, oils, salves, and so forth. This will give you an idea of what each type is and whether it has an internal or external application. Then I'll go into detail about the process of making each one. I'll provide basic recipes so you can try your hand at making each product. Don't worry; it's much easier than you think! This section is important as it gives you pearls of information to be successful at making the recipes in the remainder of the book. With a little practice, you'll then be ready to make any recipe listed. After a while you may even decide to adapt the recipes to your preference and need.

The next chapter describes sixty herbs that are an essential part of anyone's herbal medicine cabinet. While I'll be referencing many different herbs throughout the book, I passionately believe that if you choose just twenty herbs and get to know them well, you will have all the medicine you need. I've provided you with descriptions of sixty here as some will prove to be allies, and some won't. Once you begin using herbs, you'll naturally be drawn toward certain ones. This is your body's way of telling you which herbs it prefers.

We take herbs for two main reasons. One is to help remedy a symptom we are experiencing acutely, and the second is to attempt to create a shift in the body from imbalance to balance. I will refer to these two types throughout the book as acute or chronic conditions. An acute symptom refers to things like a sprained ankle or simple headache. Examples of chronic conditions are inflammation from an old injury, longstanding digestive imbalance, or hormone dysregulation.

One question frequently asked about the recipes is: How much do I take? If you are experiencing an acute situation, dosing frequently is more important than dosing in large quantities. Frequent dosing of small amounts sends a powerful message of consistency to the problem at hand that it needs to change. Dosing 1 or 2 dropperfuls of tincture or 1 cup of tea *every 2 to 3 hours* is best for acute dosing. Yes, every 2 to 3 hours. This gives the body a consistent bump of support to strengthen the system and help it regain balance.

For a chronic condition, take a small dose for a period of time, 4 to 12 weeks depending on the condition, to work with the body to create a sustained physical change. Typically the dose is 1 dropperful of tincture 2 to 3 times per day, or 2 to 3 cups of tea a day. Common dosing times are morning and night or morning, midday, and night. Think of it this way. If you've experienced chronic constipation for years, how long do you think it will take to heal the cause of what started that problem? One day? One week? Most likely not. Give it time. Herbs generally work to restore function and integrity of the body, which is not a quick fix. Give the herbs time to help the body return to a state of balance and the tissues the chance to return to a state of integrity and proper function. We ask a lot of our bodies. By giving your body this consistent attention, you can return it to health.

A note about quantities: All of the tea recipes will result in 4 ounces of loose tea. This is a standard amount and enough to make blending slightly easier. If you want to make a smaller amount, feel free to halve or quarter the recipe to begin. Tincture recipes will be created in quantities of 1 or 2 ounces, with 1 ounce of tincture equaling 30 milliliters of fluid, and 2 ounces, 60 milliliters. Capsule recipes will result in 200 capsules, and again you can reduce or double any recipe to fit your needs. All of the herbs called for in this book are to be used in dried form unless noted otherwise.

The best advice I can give is to dive right in. Read through all of the material and then give it a go. Try mixing a tea or applying a poultice for practice. The quickest way to learn is through experimentation, and the best way to learn about the herbs is to use them and to take note of how the remedies help you achieve acute symptom relief or a better balance of daily health.

I encourage you to try the recipes that seem appealing or relate to a condition or issue you've struggled with. You can read about herbs all day long, but until you actually use them you truly haven't learned anything! Just like learning anything new, using herbs for the first time can feel scary or bring up feelings of uncertainty, both of which are completely normal. The first time I tried to blend a tea, it was so bitter I had to laugh and throw it out. Expect to experience a trial-and-error period until you have a foundation underneath you.

# TYPES OF PREPARATIONS, USES, & BASIC DOSAGES FOR ADULTS

| PREPARATION | TARGETS | CHRONIC OR TONIC DOSAGE | ACUTE DOSAGE |
|---|---|---|---|
| capsule | various conditions | 2 capsules 1 or 2 times a day | 2 or 3 capsules 3 or 4 times a day |
| essential oil blend | various conditions | typically used for acute conditions | 1 to 5 drops as needed |
| flower essence blend | emotional and psychological health | 4 drops 4 times a day | 4 drops 4 times a day |
| fomentation | sprains, strains, pain, broken bones | typically used for acute conditions | enough to saturate a cloth slightly larger than affected area, applied 1 to 3 times a day for 20 minutes |
| herbal oil | skin conditions, pain, colic, lymph congestion, soreness, overall anxiety | enough to cover affected area, applied 1 to 3 times a day | enough to cover affected area, applied 1 to 3 times a day |
| medicinal tea | all physical conditions | 2 to 3 cups a day for 4 to 12 weeks | 1 cup every 2 to 3 hours as needed |
| poultice | stings, wounds, broken bones, sprains, skin conditions | typically used for acute conditions | enough to cover affected area, applied 1 or 2 times a day |
| salve | burns, cuts, scrapes, stress, pain | typcially used for acute conditions | enough to cover affected area, applied repeatedly until pain ceases |
| spray | blue moods, emotional conditions, inflammation, cuts, sore throat | typically used for acute conditions | spritz as needed or 1 to 2 sprays for physical conditions |
| suppository | vaginal dryness or pain, hemorrhoids, lower bowel laxity | typically used for acute conditions | 1 suppository 1 to 3 times a day |
| syrup | colds and coughs, headaches, upset stomach, hair and scalp conditions | typically used for acute conditions | 1 to 2 teaspoons 1 to 3 times a day |
| tincture | all physical conditions | 1 dropperful 2 to 3 times a day for 4 to 12 weeks | 1 to 2 dropperfuls every 2 to 3 hours as needed |
| wash | skin conditions, eye infections, wounds, post partum | typically used for acute conditions | 1 quart used 1 or 2 times a day |

A final note: this book is focused on recipes for those who want to make their own medicine. If you'd rather not do it yourself but want the end result of one of the recipes listed, you can always call your local herb shop to have them blend the recipe for you.

## KEY KITCHEN SUPPLIES

Here are some things you'll want to have on hand for preparing the recipes. Before you begin, sterilize all your cookware and storage containers to reduce the risk of bacterial and fungal contamination. Use the sterile mode in your dishwasher or place the items in boiling water. All your storage containers should be thoroughly dry before use. This little tip will help to ensure that your medicine lasts longer and stays fresher.

- aluminum foil
- baking dish
- calculator
- cheesecloth
- coffee filters
- coffee or nut grinder
- cooking brush or paintbrush
- cooking thermometer
- crockpot
- fine mesh strainers, small, medium, and large

- funnels, small, medium, and large
- glass containers, quart-size with secure lids
- mason jars, pint and quart size
- measuring cups, small, medium, and large
- mixing bowls
- mixing spoons
- muddling bar
- notebook
- packing rod
- pencil

- percolation vessel
- plastic sandwich bags
- rocks or paperweights
- rubber bands
- saucepan, stainless steel or ceramic
- shot glass
- soaking basin
- stockpot, stainless steel or ceramic
- Vitamix blender
- waxed paper

# Capsules

I've been amazed throughout my years as an herbalist by my customers' love of taking pills. Capsules are easy, convenient, and travel well. They also have no taste, which seems to be a big plus for many people. I also think because the supplement market is now mainstream that taking capsules and tablets is widely accepted as normal, and they are easier for many people to keep around than herbal tinctures and salves. While capsules and tablets are accessible and easy to transport, they are not always the best option. Anyone who is experiencing digestive imbalance, for example, might not be able to reap capsules' full benefit if they already have an inability to break food down properly. This can be due to a lack of digestive enzymes, digestive tract inflammation, or perhaps the material used to contain the capsule or bind the tablet. I encourage my patients to consider other modes of medicine transmission when the digestive system is challenged. There is nothing worse then wasting money on something you are hoping will work but that your body isn't able to utilize.

One thing is for sure, though—herbal capsules are extremely easy to make. You really do want to use herbal powder, as this will make the whole process much easier and quicker. You can grind the dried herb, but unless you've got an amazing herb grinder that can really get it to a powder level, I suggest purchasing prepared herb powder. Then you need to choose between two capsule materials: gelatin and vegetable glycerin. Gelatin is cheaper, but I prefer the natural substance of vegetable glycerin. The other thing to be aware of is that empty capsules come in varying sizes: 0 (the smallest), 00, and 000 (the largest). To help you visualize, my daughter calls 000 capsules "horse pills."

If you want to create a blend of different herbs for yourself, write out your blend and determine the proportions of each herb. Weigh them out and mix together before encapsulating.

# Essential Oil Blends

Essential oils, which can be blended together or added to an herbal formula, are another way in which plants can offer healing. Essential oils are derived through extraction by one of the following methods: steam distillation, water distillation, solvent extraction, enfleurage, cold press extraction, or $CO_2$ extraction. These methods basically pull out the oils of the plant, and most yield both water and essential oil. The essential oil sits on top of the water, which after processing is called a hydrosol. The oil contains specific medicinal constituents, and the hydrosol (which smells lovely but has a lighter scent

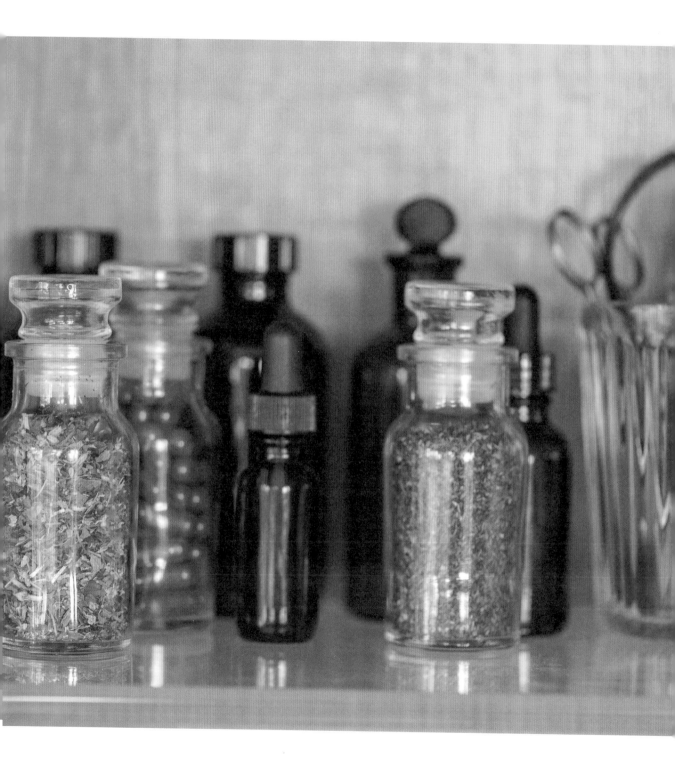

than the oil) has medicinal properties as well, but these are typically limited to the water-soluble aspects of the plant's constituents.

Some of the recipes in this book direct you to add essential oils to other ingredients for salves or herbal oils, and other recipes tell how to create essential oil blends targeting specific conditions. For blends consisting only of essential oils, essential oil quantities are indicated in milliliters since the typical essential oil bottle is 5 or 10 milliliters. If the essential oil blend involves using a carrier oil, the measurements are in drops of essential oil and ounces of carrier oil. Always use pure therapeutic essential oils in your healing recipes and be sure to keep the caps on the bottles. A pure essential oil will evaporate if the cap is left off. Read the ingredients to make sure your oils are not adulterated with carrier oils, fragrance, or perfume. The few exceptions would be the exotic essential oils such as rose, neroli, and jasmine. These are often purchased in 5- or 10-percent dilutions to make them affordable.

Essential oils can be used in many ways, but I typically don't recommend applying them directly to the skin, as they can be quite caustic. If you want to use an essential oil topically, first dilute it with olive, apricot, or coconut oil. Some essential oils, such as oregano, should never be used in direct contact with the skin. They are best added to a vaporizer or essential oil diffuser so that you are breathing in very small amounts. Some essential oils are also beneficial in a bath or as one or two drops on your pillow. And please keep in mind that essential oils are very toxic to most animals, especially cats.

## Flower Essence Blends

While herbal medicine focuses primarily on the physical health of the human body, flower essences work subtly to balance our emotional layers. Repeatedly experiencing emotions such as fear, anger, or grief can divert us from making healthy choices and can also negatively affect us on a physical level. Working with our emotions with the help of flower essences can lead to overall health on multiple levels. We can put together a custom blend to help us with the emotional and mental challenges we're facing at any given time.

Flower essences are energetic imprints of the life force of plants that interact with our spiritual essences, helping to evoke specific qualities within us. Specific flower essences have affinities for particular emotions or blockage patterns, discovered through research and study. The Flower Essence Society (flowersociety.org) in California has been conducting research since 1979 and is the leading authority. The organization offers endless resources as well as classes and certifications, should you wish to learn more.

# Fomentations

A fomentation is a strong herbal brew, similar to a wash, applied by soaking a cotton cloth in it and then placing the cloth on or wrapping it around the affected area. Heat is often added to help drive the herbs into the skin. Fomentations are perfect for applying to body parts that move or are not conducive to sitz baths or washes.

One of my favorite uses for fomentations is with my patients after any type of body treatment, whether it be acupuncture, massage, or an adjustment. Ending the appointment by placing a warm fomentation on the area worked on really sets the patient up for a good day. In a clinic I used to work at, we had a fomentation warming throughout the day so it was ready to use. The combination of herbs gave the clinic an aroma that evoked healing, and the patients loved the fomentation as it created a sense of calm, relaxation, and closure at the end of the visit.

For strains and sprains, a fomentation is an excellent first-line treatment. Areas like knees and elbows are perfect candidates for fomentations, as they are difficult to soak. Making a lavender and black cohosh fomentation for the nape of the neck can do wonders for headaches and stress. The next time loved ones are showing strain on their face or with their body language, surprise them with a fomentation treat.

# Liniments

Liniments are topical applications that can increase blood circulation and promote healing. Liniments are applied on unbroken skin and often used for sore muscles, aches, and pains. They differ from fomentations in that the solution is made with a solvent like isopropyl alcohol, witch hazel, or vinegar. Liniments penetrate and evaporate quickly on the skin's surface, but their actions can have lasting effects. A few liniment recipes are given in the book but are varied enough that I won't give a basic recipe here.

# Herbal Oils

Many people I speak with confuse herbal oils with essential oils. To be clear, an herbal oil for our purposes is an herb-infused oil, most often olive oil, that can be used topically in that form or as the base of another herbal product such as a salve, a lotion, or a cream. An essential oil is a distilled product. Both are wonderful, but they are very different from one another. Herbal oils are yet another way to use herbs topically.

You may be asking yourself at this point: When would I use an oil versus a salve or a wash? Knowing what you are treating is the first step and so is understanding the qualities of the different herbal applications. Oils and salves are both wonderful for softening, soothing, and healing skin. They are great at pulling tissues together and treating the superficial layers as well as acting as a medium to carry things slightly deeper into the body. Oil is naturally absorbed through the skin, so if it has been infused with healing herbs, the oil-soluble constituents of the herb are absorbed as well. Oils are more readily absorbed into the body than lotions. Lotions often have additional ingredients that help them sit atop the skin, whereas oils drive into deeper skin levels. But an oil-based application is not always indicated. One example is with poison ivy or oak. With a poison ivy or oak outbreak on the skin, the oil in the plant is what causes the discomfort. Using an oil-based application will only provoke and spread the condition. When you need to cool down, flush, or soak the skin, a wash is indicated. As another example, using healing oils on the perineum may be helpful, but it prefers the cooling action of a water-based application.

Herbal oils are the base of many other herbal products including salves, lotions, creams, and lip balms. Making and having a couple of herbal oils on hand allows you the freedom to whip up something when you need it or when you are looking for a fun activity on a rainy day. I prefer to make oils with fresh plant material, but dried herbs can also be used in most cases. Making oils with fresh plants generates a yearlong ongoing cycle of herbal oil production based on the plants coming up or in bloom. As I'm writing this, the mullein flowers are making their appearance and I've just made a fresh batch of mullein flower oil. Seeing the bright yellow flowers submerged in olive oil as sunshine passes through the jar on my windowsill is something that brings me peace and joy each day.

While you can make most herbal oils with fresh or dried material, some can only be processed fresh: arnica flowers, mullein flowers, and St. John's wort flowers. When using fresh material I favor the folk method, or the herbalist way as I prefer to call it. Get a jar and fill it three quarters of the way full with your plant material. Don't pack the herb too tightly or the oil can't get through and around it all. Fill the jar to the top with olive oil, close it, and set it in the sun. A consistent temperature of at least 75 to 80 degrees F is best. Shake it daily and keep an eye out for water precipitate. If it looks murky on the bottom, that usually is water precipitate and you can use a turkey baster to draw it out as needed. You can also dump the entire contents into a saucepan and gently heat it for 5 minutes, and then put it back in the jar and continue sun steeping. Two weeks is the standard amount of time for sun steeping.

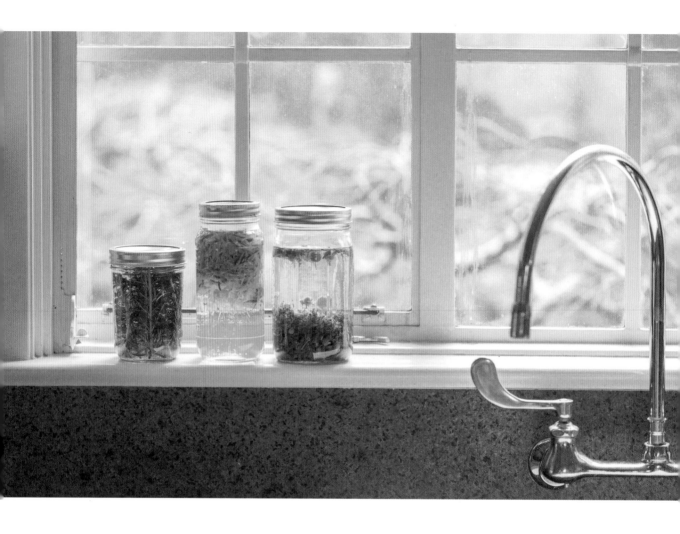

If you don't have consistent sun or are using dried herbs, the oven method will work. Place your herbs in a glass baking pan and add enough oil to cover the herbs 1 or 2 inches deep. Turn your oven on low, 170 to 200 degrees F, and bake the mixture for 4 to 6 hours. Keep an eye on it and ensure your oven isn't too hot. Stirring it from time to time is good too. Herbal oils made this way often end up with the herbs crispy and burnt looking. This is normal, as long as your oven wasn't too hot and your oil is not burnt. Strain into a glass jar and store the oil in a dark, cool place.

# Medicinal Teas

Herbal teas, so often associated with specific flavors rather than specific medicinal effects, are unsung herbal heroes able to create significant physiological changes in the body. It's hard not to say that every herb tea has medicinal value, in fact. Something considered as benign as chamomile tea can have significant effects on the body. I've seen women who regularly drink chamomile tea experience decreased menstrual cramping and more regulated cycles. Some people have a ritual of drinking peppermint tea after dinner simply because they like the taste and realize it cleanses the palate; they may not know that it became an after-dinner tradition because of the digestive support it offers.

Medicinal teas made from herbal blends can be brewed by the cup as needed or in batches designed to provide one day's worth of medicine. I don't recommend making herbal tea in larger batches, as many of the herbs don't keep well after a day or two. Even in the refrigerator, some herbs like slippery elm bark or marshmallow root will sour the tea once it is made or impart a bitter flavor. A batch is 1 quart or roughly 3 10-ounce cups of tea. You can make a quart of tea one of two ways. Both are equally fine; it's just a matter of preference and whether you need something immediately or can prepare ahead of time.

# Poultices

I've always considered a poultice one of the most primitive yet effective ways to use herbs for healing. By definition a poultice is a soft, damp mass of material, typically plant material or plant material mixed with flour, applied to the body to relieve soreness and inflammation. It's applied in a thick layer and kept in place with a cloth. You may have seen recommendations to add heat, but I haven't found that to be necessary in order for the poltice to be effective. Many times the natural heat of the body is sufficient.

You might have had a grandmother who sautéed onions and ginger whenever you had a cold. Not to eat, mind you, but to then mix with flour and stuff into an old sock to apply to your throat and neck. When I was a kid this was torture, but I really cannot think of a time when it didn't eventually put me to sleep and greatly reduce whatever cold was ailing me.

In both Western and Chinese herbalism, making an herb cake from fresh or dried herbs and applying it directly to the skin is common. Taking the herb, mixing it with a bit of hot water to open it up, and then placing it on the affected area is the easiest way. If you are out and about and don't have hot water, simply sticking the fresh herb into your mouth to macerate it works great too. Just ensure it's an herb that is safe to eat. The saliva actually does a good job of keeping it all together so it can then be spit out and held in place on the skin. I live on a farm, and we are outside a lot and frequently get splinters. Most of the time they are easy enough to pull out, but sometimes a poultice is needed to soften the surrounding skin so I can get ahold of the splinter. Using drawing herbs such as plantain and comfrey leaf can turn tears into smiles with my kids as we pick the leaves and chew to our hearts' content before spitting on each other. Letting the poultice sit for as little as five minutes usually draws out the tip of the splinter just enough to grasp it.

Practice making poultices in the following way so you are confident in their use when you need them. With dried or fresh herbs, mash just enough in a small bowl with a splash of hot water to cover the affected area. If using fresh, cut or tear into small pieces before mashing. Mash until the mixture has a pastelike consistency. Once it has cooled a bit, apply to the affected area. If you can relax for 15 to 20 minutes, do so and hold still so the poultice stays in place. If you need to be on the go, wrap with sterile gauze or cover with a large Band-Aid. You can leave the poultice on as long as it seems helpful, but keeping it clean and refreshing it regularly is necessary.

## Salves

A salve, which is applied topically, can also be referred to as an ointment, a balm, an emollient, or sometimes a cream. Its base is typically beeswax, although many people have begun switching to vegan options such as candelilla wax and shea butter. By infusing herbs into oil and then adding the wax, you get a semisolid substance that can be spread onto the skin when and where it's needed. Used throughout history on animals and people, salves historically had bases of bear grease, lard, and other animal fats.

A salve is applied to soothe the body. Dabbing a bit of salve onto whatever is ailing you is an easy way to introduce herbs into your life. Most of us cannot get through a week without some small paper cut, hangnail, burn, or bug bite. Yes, all these will heal on their own, but why not offer yourself a touch of relief? Is a heavy workload causing you some muscle tension? Apply a bit of relief salve to relax the tension. Herbal medicine is just as much about learning to take the time to care for yourself as it is about healing specific symptoms.

Once you've decided which condition you're trying to remedy with a salve, you need to decide if you'd like the salve to be scented or not. Adding essential oils to the salve will help it smell good and also provide extra healing potential and a longer shelf life. Doing a bit of research regarding essential oils will really pay off in the end. With each salve recipe

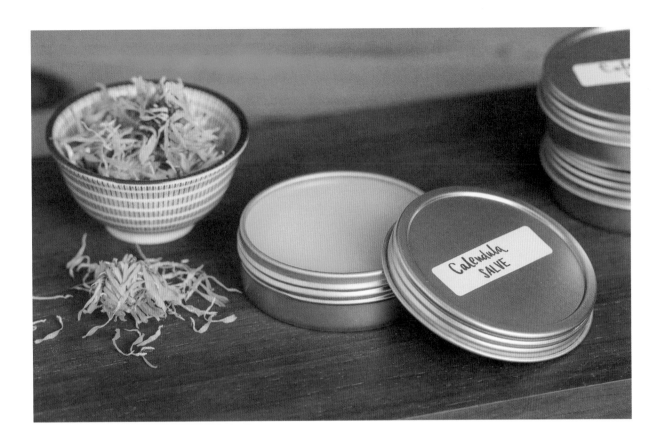

later in the book, I indicate specific essential oils that will complement the healing process. That being said, if you plan to use your salve quickly and prefer it to be unscented, that is fine too. Just keep it in a cool place for longevity.

All you need in order to make a salve is a medicinal herbal oil, beeswax, and a container to put it in. It really is that simple. When using a salve, a little goes a long way but you always want to cover the area completely. Having a little bit sit on top of the injured area is just fine—it acts as a natural bandage.

## Sprays

Sprays are easy to create and use. Just a spritz here and a spritz there can quickly shift emotions, calm inflammation, soothe a cut, or transform the smell of a room.

# Suppositories

Suppositories are another way to deliver herbal medicine. These small, semisoft cone- or dome-shaped preparations, usually with a cocoa butter base, are great for targeting treatment to the vaginal or lower intestinal/anal regions of the body. I often recommend them for vaginal dryness or pain as well as for hemorrhoids or laxity of the lower bowel. Using suppository molds makes the whole process very simple.

# Syrups

The base of any syrup is a strong herbal tea that has been simmered and reduced to create a concentrated brew. This is then combined with honey or sugar and voilà, you have herbal syrup. It's another example of the ease of making herbal medicines. If the medicine from an herb is water soluble, you can make an herbal syrup.

You may be familiar with elderberry syrup, as it hit the mainstream several years ago. High in antioxidants and with antiviral properties, it's a great addition to any household's medicine cabinet. And of course most of us have experienced cough syrup at some point in our lives. But syrups aren't just for colds and flus. You can also make headache syrup, mineral syrup, hair tonic syrup, and kids' tummy tamer syrup. The extra bonus is that herbal syrups typically taste delicious and are an easy way to get even the pickiest of palettes to try herbal medicine.

The question that typically arises here is: If I'm using leaves and flowers, won't the simmering hurt the final product? Honestly, I don't have an answer here. I often think of Susun Weed when I'm asked this question. In one conversation we had, we were discussing eating our greens verses taking vitamins and herbs to get our calcium. We agreed that eating greens is by far superior to getting the nutrient in other ways. I like to cook greens lightly, but Susun, like my mother, is big on cooking greens way down, reasoning that this allows for complete breakdown of the plant material so it can be readily assimilated in the body. I grew up with mushy vegetables, and once I began studying nutrition I was thrilled to learn that light cooking kept many nutrients intact. So you can see my dilemma. To cook or not to cook down? There are good reasons either way; it just depends on what you're hoping to get. So for syrups, when you're trying to create a thick, concentrated base, cooking the herbs down on low heat makes sense to me.

## Tinctures

A tincture is a solution created by soaking an herb in alcohol to extract its healing properties, resulting in a medicine that can be taken by mouth. While tinctures can be made in mediums other than alcohol, such as vinegar or vegetable glycerin, alcohol is the most commonly used. The advantages of using alcohol are that it works with almost any plant (unlike vinegar or glycerin), you can formulate the optimal alcohol percentage in which a plant's constituents will extract (the plant's solubility range), and the alcohol base allows for sublingual transmission, meaning the medicine will bypass the digestive system and go more directly into the bloodstream—particularly helpful when medicine is needed to treat an acute situation. When I'm having menstrual cramps, for example, I take a tincture so it begins to work right away instead of taking a capsule and having

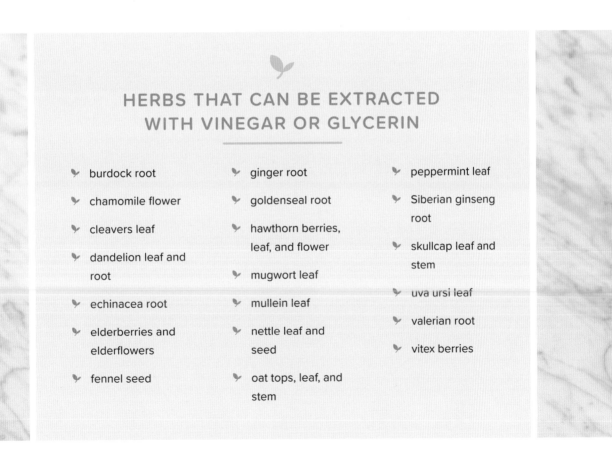

### HERBS THAT CAN BE EXTRACTED WITH VINEGAR OR GLYCERIN

- burdock root
- chamomile flower
- cleavers leaf
- dandelion leaf and root
- echinacea root
- elderberries and elderflowers
- fennel seed

- ginger root
- goldenseal root
- hawthorn berries, leaf, and flower
- mugwort leaf
- mullein leaf
- nettle leaf and seed
- oat tops, leaf, and stem

- peppermint leaf
- Siberian ginseng root
- skullcap leaf and stem
- uva ursi leaf
- valerian root
- vitex berries

to wait 40 minutes. A tincture definitely has an alcohol flavor, so if you cannot tolerate that, refer to the sidebar to see whether the herbs you'd like to use can be extracted with apple cider vinegar or vegetable glycerin.

To make a tincture, I recommend starting small. There is no need to create a quart of burdock tincture for yourself unless you want a lifetime supply or are planning to share it with your friends. Use 1- to 4-ounce jars to begin with. Start with making a simple—a one-herb tincture. You can use either fresh or dried herbs when making a tincture, and for practicality's sake I'll only describe the folk tincture-making method in this book. If you are looking for other tincture-making options, please refer to my previous book, *The Herbal Apothecary.*

If using fresh leaves, flowers, roots, or bark, cut up the fresh material into small pieces before putting it into your extracting jar. Fill the jar halfway with your herb of choice (although I often put in more than that for good measure). When using dried herbs, fill the jar a fifth to a third full. Then add vodka, filling the jar to the top, and close with a tight-fitting lid. Vodka works well because it consists of 40 to 50 percent alcohol, which makes it a good fit for most herbs. The higher up the vodka is on the shelf at the liquor store, the better the quality, which equates with better taste. (Taste is hugely important to me as the better it tastes, the more likely I am to take it. When a tincture tastes like burning fuel, I tend to struggle with the desire to take it.) Next, add a label to the jar. Put the name of the herb, today's date, and the date 4 weeks from now. Give it a good shake and set it somewhere where you will remember to shake it daily. The shaking is important, as it agitates the plant material to break down and release the plant's constituents. Watch over the next 4 weeks as the color shifts and changes. This a favorite phase for me. I often feel very connected to the plant during this phase, as my intention is with it almost daily.

After the 4 weeks, strain the tincture twice through a fine-mesh sieve or a cheesecloth-lined colander to ensure all particulate matter is out. Store the tincture in a dark amber or blue dropper bottle with a proper name label and date. To maintain potency, tinctures are best kept out of direct sunlight, in a cool pantry or cupboard. While I don't believe in a shelf life for tinctures that have been stored properly, you can safely consider them viable for 3 to 5 years.

Sometimes I recommend using already prepared and purchased tinctures to make tincture blends. In these cases, the measurements are in milliliters to correspond to how purchased tinctures are packaged.

# Washes

I use the term *herbal wash* to describe a single herb or a blend of herbs used to bathe, wash, or soak a part of the body. A great example is my eczema wash at Fettle. Eczema ranges in severity from mild to debilitating, but any form is uncomfortable. Itching, cracking of skin, dryness, and pain can all accompany this condition. Steeping a blend of cooling, anti-inflammatory, and emollient herbs and allowing the affected body part to soak in the cooled-down brew often provides much-needed relief.

I've successfully used washes for pink eye, cradle cap, and various other skin conditions. I also put sitz baths into this category. Sitz baths are an old nature cure technique derived from the German *sitzbad*, meaning a bath (*bad*) in which one sits (*sitzen*). They are often used after labor to heal the vagina and perineum and also helpful with hemorrhoid healing and relief. It is a deeper submersion of the bottom, pelvis, and hip regions. As you can imagine, the herbal wash targets the tissues in need, but it also works to gently move circulation and lymph channels in the area. While you can do a sitz bath in a shallow bathtub, you will find it difficult to get the herb-to-water ratio right. I prefer to use a plastic washbasin because you get the greatest surface area covered with a concentrated medicinal brew.

Even stronger than a medicinal-strength tea, an herbal wash is made with a recommended 6 tablespoons of herb per quart or 3 tablespoons per pint. I also suggest steeping the herbs for 1 or 2 hours before using the wash. You can steep overnight if you prefer and reheat if necessary. Soaking for 20 to 60 minutes is best.

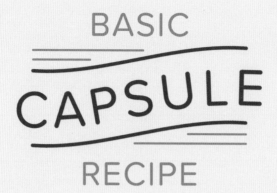

# BASIC CAPSULE RECIPE

**2 ounces powdered herb(s)**
**200 empty capsules**

Place the powdered herbs in the capsules using either the homestyle method or a capsule maker. For homestyle, follow these steps:

1   Put the herbal powder in a bowl. Approximately 2 ounces will make 200 capsules, give or take depending on the capsule size.

2   Separate a capsule and scoop herbal powder from the bowl into each side of the capsule. It's like a diving-for-herb-powder experience. Your fingers will get a little dirty.

3   Close the capsule. Careful not to overfill or you won't be able to close it.

*continued . . .*

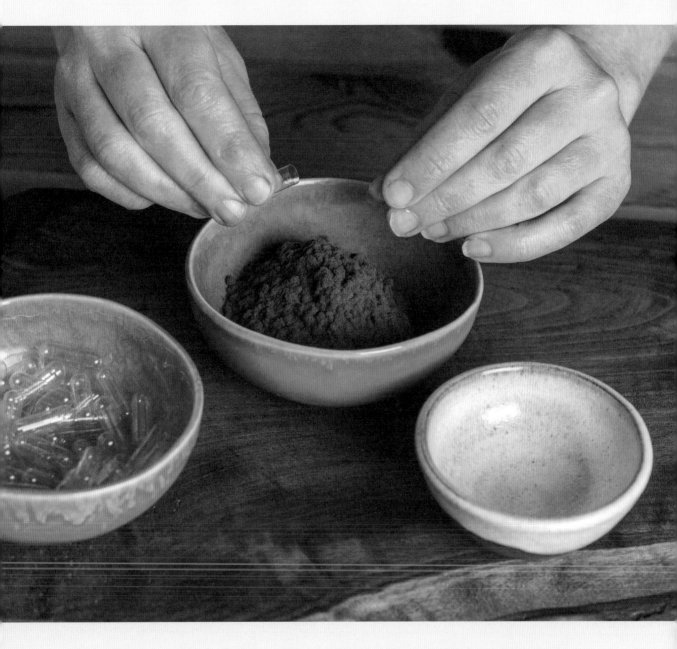

▲ Put powdered herbal material in a bowl and scoop the powder into the capsule halves. Then close the capsule.

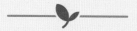

If you'd rather invest in a capsule maker, such as a Cap-M-Quik, they are very easy to use and you can make 200 capsules very quickly. Instructions are included, but basically you put the bottom part (the larger piece) of the capsule into the tray and then pour the powder onto the tray. You use the spreading tool to disperse the powder evenly and then gently tap it down. Once the capsules are filled, you lower the tray. The bottom parts of the capsules are exposed and all you need to do is stick on the tops.

At my herb shop, Fettle Botanic Supply & Counsel, I package my capsule products in paper cannisters to keep the costs down and the price reflective of what you are purchasing, which is the medicine. At home I recommend you store your capsules in a glass jar away from heat and sunlight. The closed glass jar helps to keep them fresh for a long time.

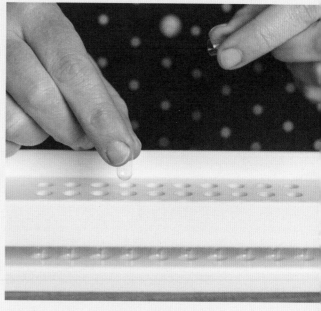

1 · Put the capsule bottoms into the raised tray.

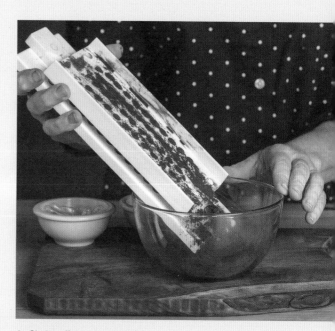

4 · Shake off the extra powder.

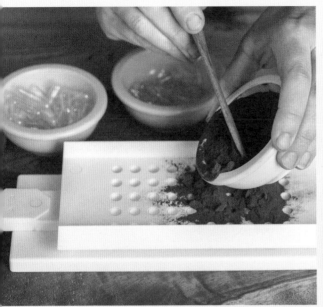

2 · Pour the powder onto the tray.

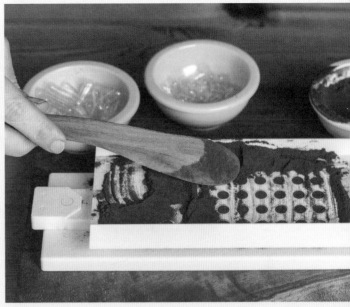

3 · Use the spreading tool to disperse and tap down.

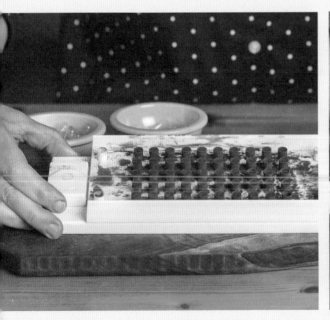

5 · Lower the tray.

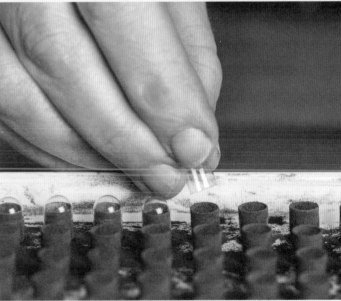

6 · Stick on the tops.

# BASIC
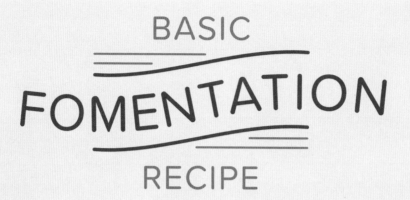
# FOMENTATION
## RECIPE

**6 tablespoons fresh or dried herbs**
**1 quart water**

Mix the herbs with the water and steep one or two hours. Strain the herbs out and gently warm up in a saucepan on the stove on low. Soak a cotton cloth in the pan, wring it out, and apply to affected area.

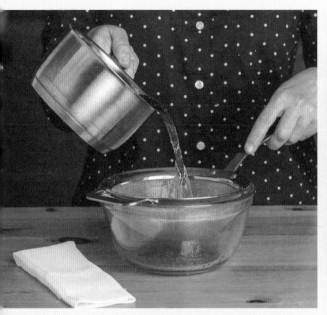

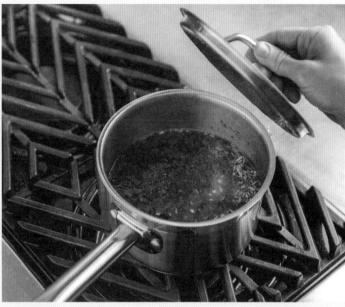

1 · Mix herbs with water in a container and steep for one or two hours. Strain herbs and pour into saucepan.

2 · Gently warm on low.

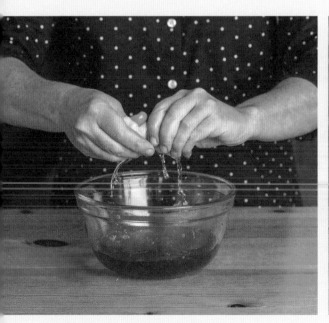

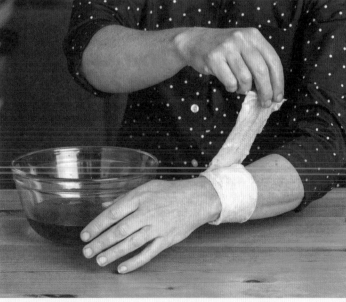

3 · Soak cloth in warm fomentation and wring out.

4 · Apply to affected area.

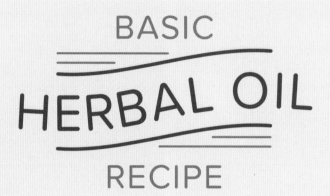

# BASIC HERBAL OIL RECIPE

**fresh or dried herbs**

**olive oil**

FOR FRESH HERBS, loosely fill a pint jar three quarters full of the herb and fill it to the top with olive oil. Close the lid and sun steep for 2 weeks.

FOR DRIED HERBS, put the desired amount of the herb in a small glass baking pan and cover with olive oil to a depth of 1 or 2 inches. Bake at 170 to 200 degrees F in the oven, stirring occasionally, for 4 to 6 hours. Strain into a glass jar and store in a dark, cool place.

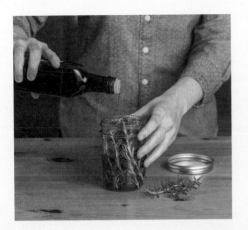

# FOR THE SUN-STEEPING METHOD:

Fill a jar three quarters full of fresh herbs, top up with olive oil, close the lid, and steep for 2 weeks in the sun.

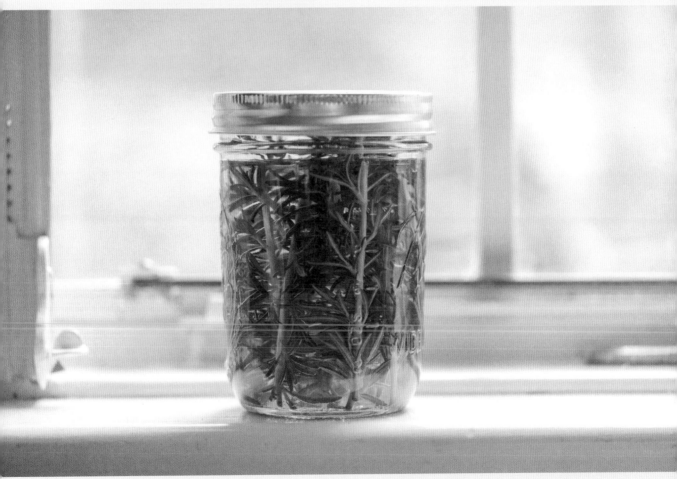

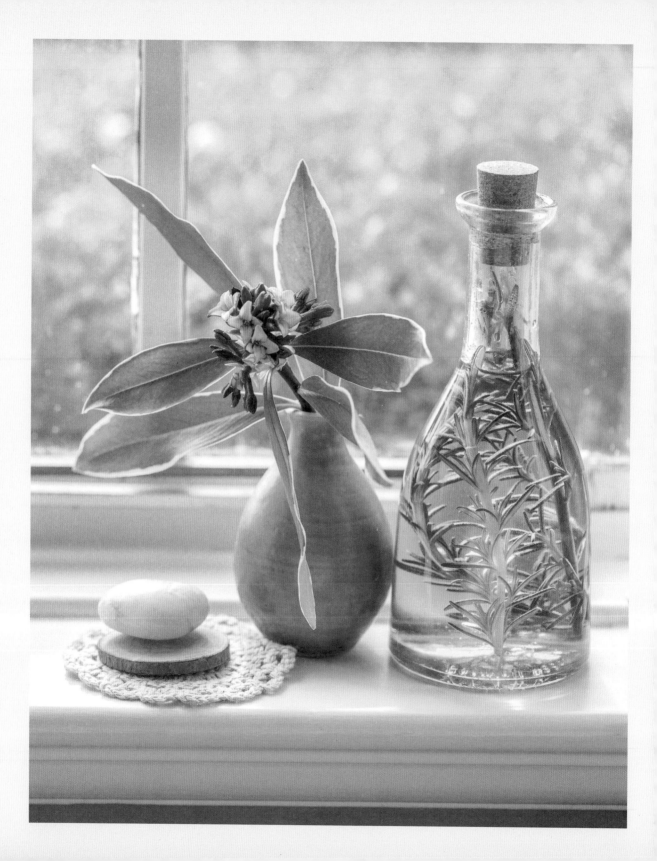

# FOR *THE* OVEN METHOD →

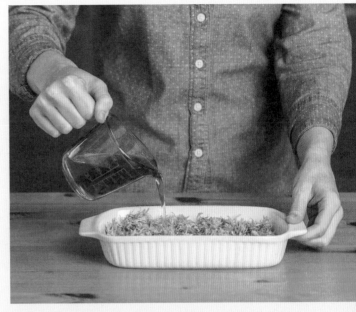

1 · Place the herbs in a glass baking pan and cover with olive oil.

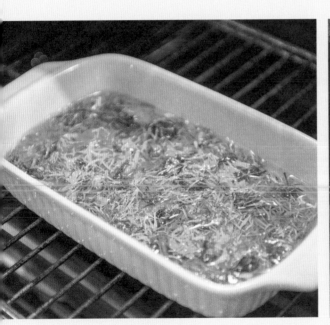

2 · Bake at 170 to 200 degrees for 4 to 6 hours.

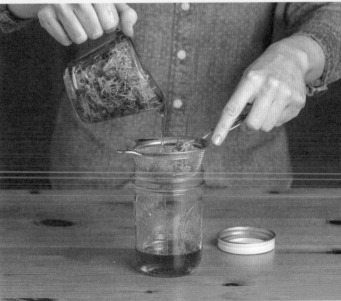

3 · Strain into a glass storage container.

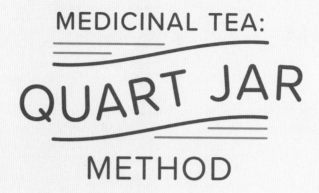

# MEDICINAL TEA: QUART JAR METHOD

Place 4 to 5 tablespoons of dried herbs in a quart jar. Set a full kettle of water on the stove and turn on the heat. Right before the water boils, or at around 200 degrees F, pull the kettle off the heat. After a while your ear will be trained to hear the almost boiling point. Pour the hot water over the herbs to almost the top of the jar. Close with the lid or place a tea towel over the top and let sit 4 hours or overnight. The hot water, combined with the longer steeping time, will work to steep all plant material types, whether leaves, roots, or flowers. Once steeping is complete, strain the tea. Divide this up into 3 cups for the day, drinking it hot or cold, depending on your mood, constitution, and personal preference.

Most often teas are steeped and drunk hot, but if a cooling effect is desired you can try drinking it cold. If you are dealing with a complaint like a phlegmy head cold, drinking it hot will aid the herbs' efforts. While most research shows drinking tea hot is more beneficial, an herb like marshmallow root is great cold to soothe bladder inflammation. And some teas such as marshmallow, slippery elm, chamomile, and blessed thistle are best steeped using cold water. These herbs have mucilage and/or bitter compounds that should be preserved and that to a small extent might be decreased with boiling water. Remember, cold-brewed tea is a natural diuretic, which means it can increase urination.

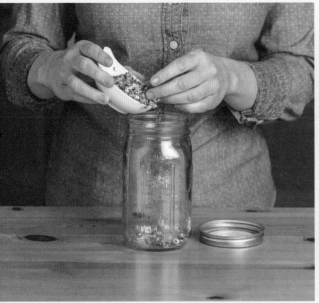

1 · Place the herbs in a quart jar.

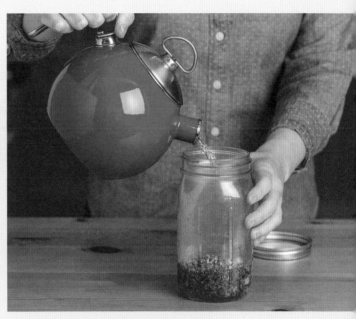

2 · Pour hot water over the herbs almost to the top.

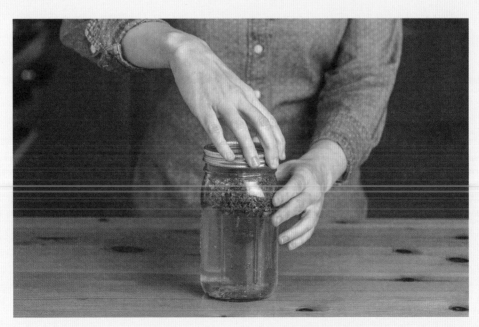

3 · Close the jar with its lid or place a tea towel over the top and allow to steep 4 hours or overnight.

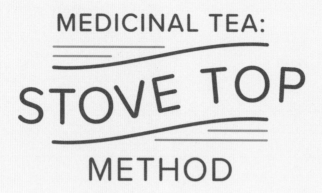

# MEDICINAL TEA: STOVE TOP METHOD

Sometimes you need a cup of medicinal tea quickly. In this case or if you prefer, you can make your medicinal tea on the stove top. With the quart jar method, it doesn't matter if you have leaves, flowers, roots, or bark, as the long duration of steeping allows all the constituents to be extracted. In the stove top method, the herb part determines the process. If you have an herbal blend that has roots and bark only, this process is quite easy. Simply put 1 quart plus ½ cup extra of water in a pot on your stove and turn on the heat. Once it begins to boil, turn it down to a simmer, add 4 to 5 tablespoons of herbs, and cover for 15 minutes. Ensure it is a light simmer. If the water is boiling, you'll lose too much of it in the process. After 15 minutes, turn off the heat and let cool slightly. Strain the tea.

If your tea consists of a combination of roots and flowers and leaves, you will need to complete an extra step. The more delicate parts of herbs such as flowers and leaves cannot tolerate high simmering heat, as it destroys their potency. Therefore, you'll complete the steps described in the previous paragraph, but once you turn off the heat, you'll add 1 more tablespoon of the herbal blend, give a quick stir, cover the pot back up, and let it steep for 10 to 15 minutes. This allows for infusion of the leaves and/or flowers into the water. Then you can strain the herbs from the water and enjoy.

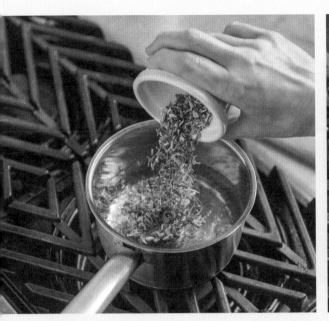

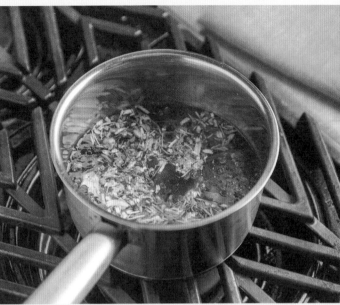

1 · Add the herbs to simmering water.

2 · Ensure tea is at a light simmer, then cover for 15 minutes.

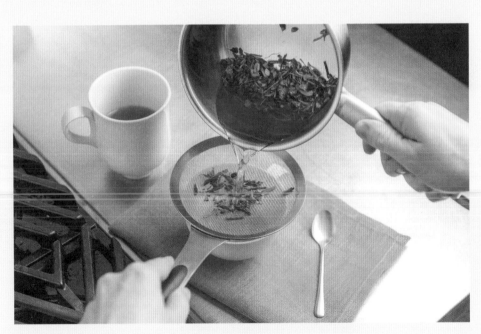

3 · Let cool slightly, strain the herbs from the water, and enjoy.

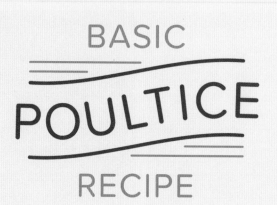

# BASIC POULTICE RECIPE

**2–5 fresh herb leaves**
**1–3 teaspoons hot water**

Dice the fresh herb leaves and place in a small bowl. Add enough hot water to mash and mix into a pastelike consistency. Apply to affected area for 15 to 20 minutes. Cover with a Band-Aid or sterile gauze wrap if you have to be on the go.

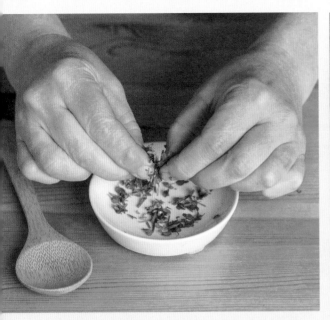

1 · Cut or tear fresh material into small pieces.

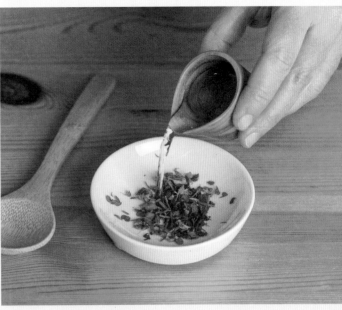

2 · Pour in a splash of hot water.

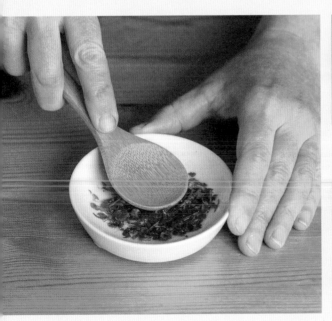

3 · Mash and mix into a paste.

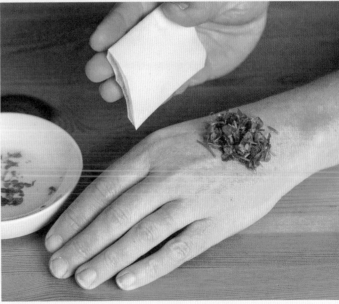

4 · Apply to affected area and wrap with sterile gauze or apply a Band-Aid.

# BASIC

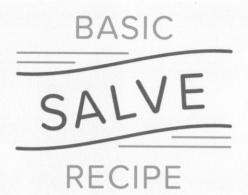

## SALVE

## RECIPE

½ cup herbal oil

½ ounce beeswax

20 drops essential oil of your choice (optional)

Gently heat the oil, add the beeswax, and stir until melted. Add essential oil if you choose. Pour the salve into a jar. Let it cool completely before putting on the lid.

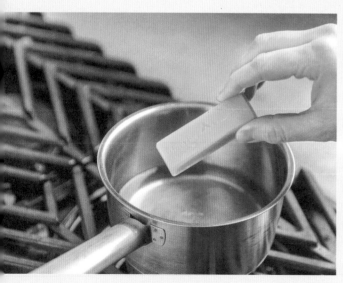

1 · Heat the oil, then add the beeswax and stir until melted. Add optional essential oils.

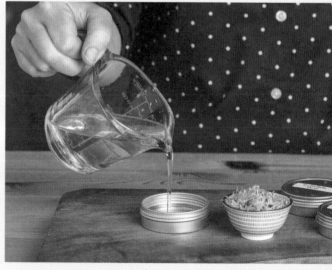

2 · Pour into a container and let cool before putting on the lid.

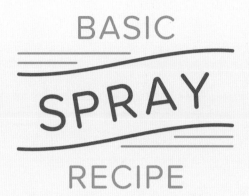

# BASIC SPRAY RECIPE

**1–2 ounces distilled water**

**10–20 drops essential oil(s) or 1 ounce herbal tincture**

Pour the water into a 2-ounce spray bottle and add your essential oil(s) or herbal tincture. Shake gently before spritzing.

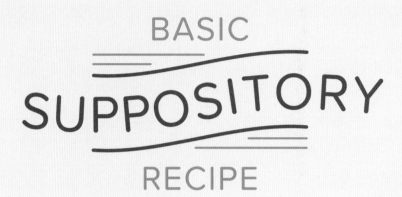

# BASIC SUPPOSITORY RECIPE

suppository mold holder

suppository molds

¼ cup cocoa butter

¼ cup coconut oil

1 tablespoon herbal oil

3 tablespoons
  powdered herb(s)

Gently heat the cocoa butter, coconut oil, and herbal oil together until blended. Next, turn off the heat, add the powdered herbs, and stir for 3 to 5 minutes. Pour into molds and put into the refrigerator to harden. Once hardened, store in the refrigerator in the molds or remove from the molds and store in a glass jar.

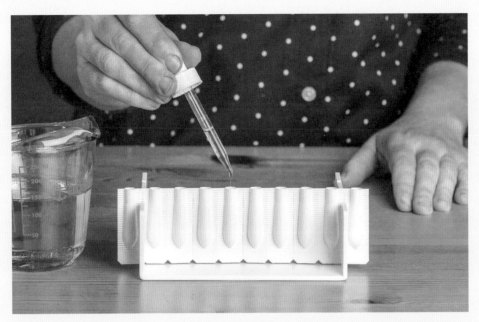

1 · Use a dropper to pour the oil and herb blend into suppository molds. Put into refrigerator to harden.

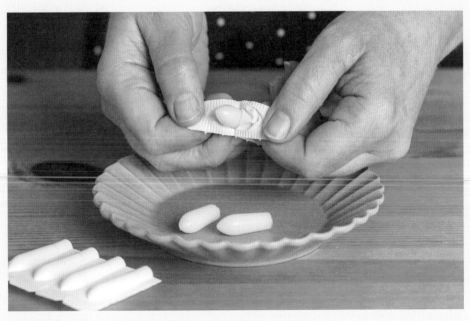

2 · Remove suppositories from the molds and refrigerate in a glass jar.

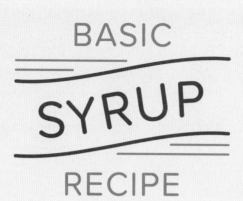

# BASIC SYRUP RECIPE

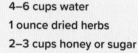

**4–6 cups water**

**1 ounce dried herbs**

**2–3 cups honey or sugar**

Bring the water to a boil in a saucepan and add the herbs. Lower the heat and simmer with the lid on or ajar until the liquid is reduced by half. Double strain the herbs from the liquid. Pour the liquid into a measuring cup to measure, then pour back into a clean saucepan and add an equal amount of honey or raw cane sugar. Gently heat on low, continuously stirring until the honey or sugar has dissolved. Allow to cool then transfer into an amber bottle. Refrigerate if you've made a large batch.

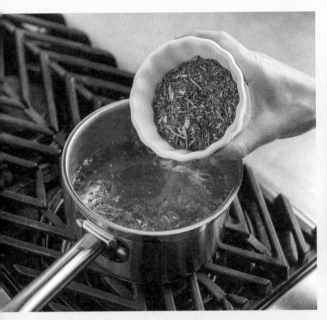

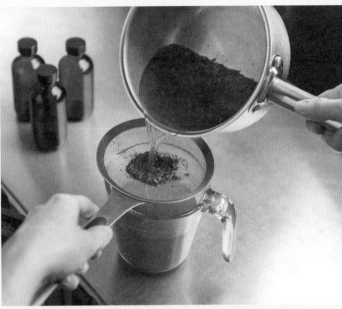

1 · Put the herbs into boiling water in a saucepan. Cover and simmer until liquid is reduced by half.

2 · Double strain the herbs from the liquid and measure volume.

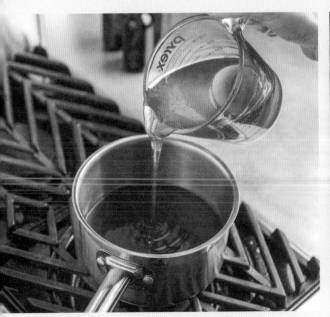

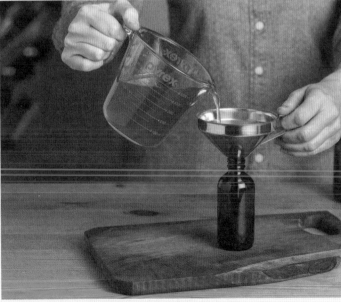

3 · Pour back into a clean saucepan and add an equal amount of honey or raw cane sugar.

4 · Allow to cool then pour into an amber bottle.

51

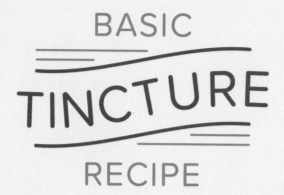

# BASIC TINCTURE RECIPE

fresh or dried herb
vodka

If the herb is fresh, cut it into small pieces. Fill a 4-ounce jar a third full with the herb and fill to the top with vodka. Close tightly and shake well. Allow to macerate (to soften by soaking) for 4 weeks in a cool, dark place, shaking daily. Strain and transfer the liquid into a dark blue or amber dropper bottle for future use.

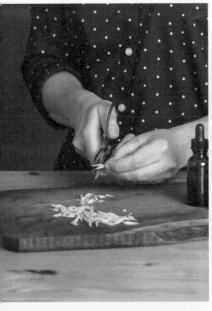
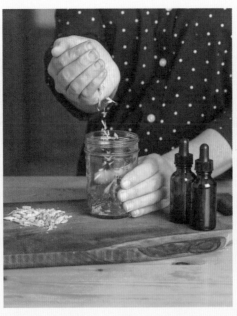
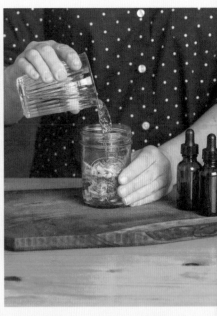

1 · Cut up fresh material into small pieces.

2 · Fill a 4-ounce jar a third full with the herb.

3 · Add vodka to fill, then close tightly and store in a cool, dark place, shaking daily.

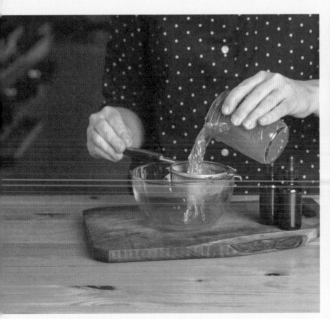
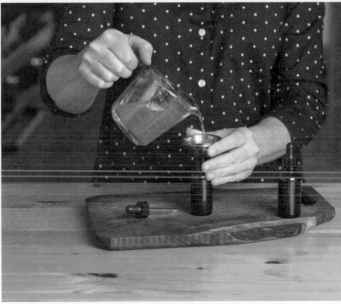

4 · Strain out the herb.

5 · Transfer to a blue or amber dropper bottle.

# BASIC WASH RECIPE

**6 tablespoons dried herb or herbal mixture**

**1 quart hot water**

Pour the hot water over the herbs and close the container with a lid. Let steep 1 or 2 hours or overnight. Strain and pour the brew into a basin. Rewarm if necessary for treatment. Soak 20 to 60 minutes.

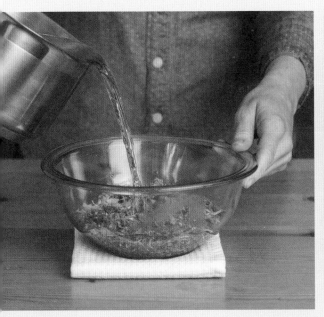

1 · Pour hot water over the herbs.

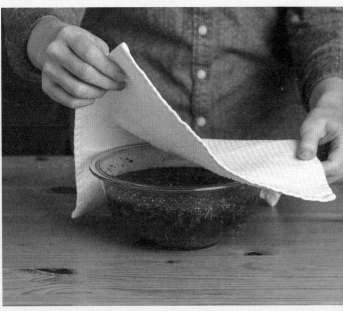

2 · Cover the container and allow to steep 1 to 2 hours or overnight.

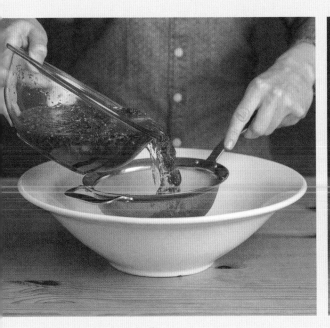

3 · Strain and pour into a basin

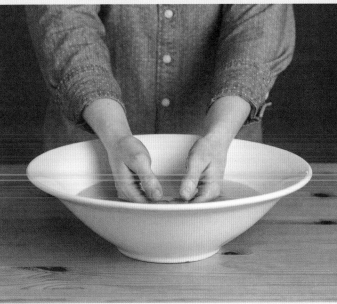

4 · Soak the affected body part.

55

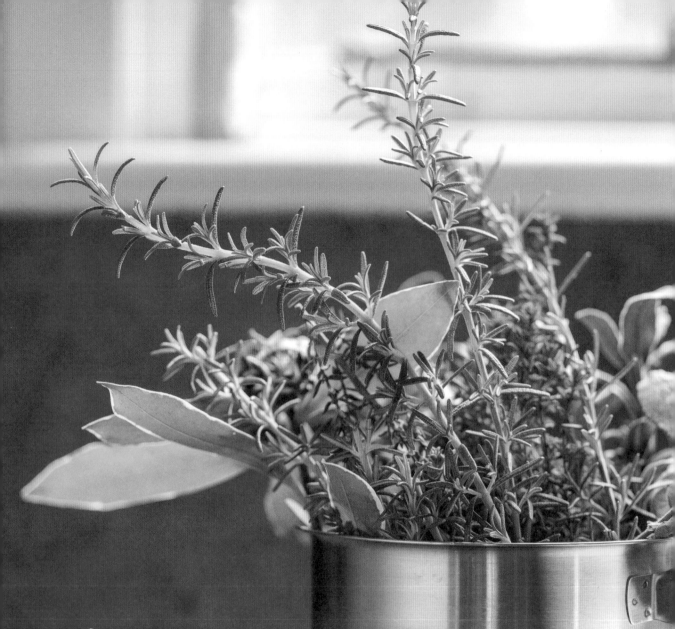

# Key Ingredients

## MUST-HAVE HERBS FOR DAY-TO-DAY USE

THE HERBS PROFILED HERE are those I recommend to create a beginner's library. These are good all-round, all-star herbs because they are readily available and generally considered safe for public consumption. Recipes using them are given in the sections of the book indicated in the "Helpful for" line in the profiles. As you read through the book, you will create your own list of herbs that call to you. Having a small, curated herbal medicinary in your home enables you to care for yourself in a unique and powerful way.

## WHERE TO GET HERBS

As you'll see, many herbs overlap in action, but not all herbs grow everywhere, hence the need to reference many options and then to learn which herbs grow in your region. You can always purchase herbs from reputable herb shops, but finding them in your local area is a fun adventure and gives new insight into the herbs. Growing your own medicinal herbs is also a rewarding experience and is more sustainable than collecting them from the wild. If you do the latter, it's called wildcrafting, and it's important to follow these rules:

- Ensure the plants have not been sprayed with pesticides.

- Ensure you are collecting the correct plant.

- Ensure the plant is not endangered from overcollecting. If it is, admire but do not collect.

- If harvesting, take only a quarter of the plant population found in the area. This ensures future generations of the plant will thrive.

- Never harvest bark from a live tree. Look for fallen branches to collect from.

- As a personal favor, I ask you to speak to the plant first before collecting. While plants are willing to share their medicine with us, it is kind to be grateful for it.

## ASHWAGANDHA

*Withania somnifera*

PARTS USED roots   HELPFUL FOR immune defense, women's health, babies and children, emotional support, travel health

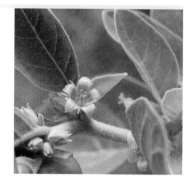

Usually in the immune defense department, this herb supports immune system health and also balances out the body, particularly the mood. I have seen ashwagandha alone uplift a patient's mood and affect after it has been taken consistently for 2 weeks. When the body feels strong and well, it is much easier to have a positive outlook.

## BLACK COHOSH

*Actaea racemosa* (also *Cimicifuga racemosa*)

PARTS USED rhizomes, roots   HELPFUL FOR day-to-day health, women's health, emotional support, elders' health

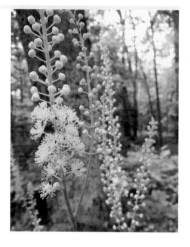

This herb, commonly thought of as a women's reproductive herb, has an amazing effect on calming the central nervous system. When someone's anxiety triggers the physical response of tremors, black cohosh should be included in the formula. I once had a patient who would begin to shake as if she were cold every time she became nervous or anxious, or thought about something worrisome. Using a nervine blend that included black cohosh made a significant improvement. As it is a smooth muscle relaxant, I often also use it to calm muscle tension.

## BURDOCK

*Arctium lappa*

PARTS USED roots   HELPFUL FOR day-to-day health, emotional support

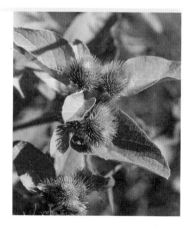

Traditionally thought of as a liver herb, burdock root offers consistent support for the detoxification process and direct healing for the lining of the stomach and its function. The root is most often used, but the leaves create mild bile stimulation and are used as a wash for poison oak/ivy. I often use burdock root for those who need more grounding in their lives, those who are scattered by too much thought or responsibility, or those whose head is always in the clouds. If your energy is perpetually up and running or you tend to live outside of your body, burdock is a good choice. Be careful using it with those who already demonstrate a depressive nature.

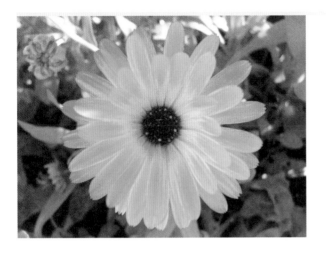

## CALENDULA

*Calendula officinalis*

PARTS USED flowers    HELPFUL FOR day-to-day health, babies and children

Nature's healing flower, Calendula is known to pull tissues together to expedite healing. Antibacterial by nature, it is a great herb to keep areas free from infection while working to heal the wound. Used internally for gastritis, menstrual pain, fever, and recurring vomiting. The bright, beautiful flowers of calendula are always a hit with little ones. And when they learn that these flowers can help heal their cuts and scrapes, things get really exciting.

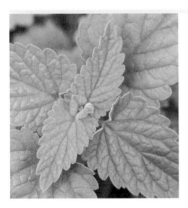

## CATNIP

*Nepeta cataria*

PARTS USED leaves    HELPFUL FOR babies and children

Not just for cats! This herb is one of the best for nervous stomach issues. When kids are young, they first learn about being in their bodies. What this means is identifying bodily sensations such as hunger, thirst, and needing to use the bathroom; then the identification of emotions begins. This is often when I see pediatric patients who complain of stomachaches. Kids are notorious for holding emotions in their tummies, and catnip is a great herbal ally to call upon in such times.

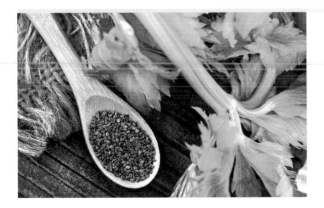

## CELERY

*Apium graveolens*

PARTS USED seeds    HELPFUL FOR emotional support

One of my go-to herbs for anxiety. I'd read about its ability to alleviate stress and particularly anxiety symptoms some years back and decided to give it a try with one of my patients, who couldn't stop her thoughts from spiraling out of control. The results were amazing. She immediately reported a sense of calm that she'd not felt in a long time.

## CHAMOMILE

*Matricaria chamomilla*

PARTS USED flowers    HELPFUL FOR babies and children, day-to-day complaints, women's health, elders' health

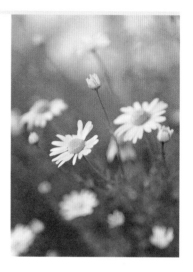

Most of us think of chamomile only for sleepy time teas, but this herb provides a lot of healing opportunity. It helps with stomach complaints, skin irritations, allergies, eye pain, menstrual irregularity, stress, hemorrhoids, toothaches, and lower back pain. This gentle flower is particularly helpful for children. Easing discomforts of the stomach and head, it can be used in teas, glycerin-based tinctures, and fomentations. It is my go-to with my little boy, who often gets angry with pain. As he is just a baby, he doesn't understand pain and it makes him very frustrated. When this occurs and he cannot be comforted by even his favorite things, using chamomile has proven very helpful.

## COLTSFOOT

*Tussilago farfara*

PARTS USED leaves    HELPFUL FOR immune defense

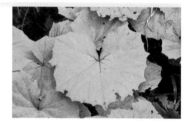

Coltsfoot is a respiratory herb that focuses on opening up breathing pathways to clear phlegm and constriction in the lungs. Antimicrobial by nature and soothing to the respiratory tract, it is excellent for dry cough and sore throat.

## COMFREY

*Symphytum officinale*

PARTS USED leaves    HELPFUL FOR day-to-day health, women's health, men's health, babies and children, travel health, elders' health

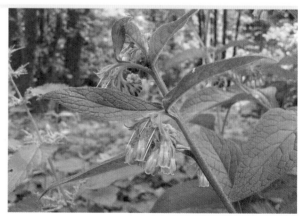

This herb grows tall and has what I refer to as fairy flowers along long stalks. With emollient, demulcent, and vulnerary properties, comfrey is a healing plant internally and externally. I use it for various skin afflictions and to soften the skin overall. Internally it seems to help almost any chronic digestive problem, most likely due to its ability to soothe and coat the stomach and intestines with its protective constituents. Highly astringent, it can help to stop bleeding and excessive discharges from the body. The leaves can be applied to broken bones to help the healing process.

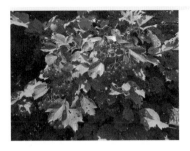

### CRAMP BARK

*Viburnum opulus*

PARTS USED bark    HELPFUL FOR day-to-day health, women's health, babies and children, travel health

Cramp bark works to relax smooth muscle. It is often used for uterine cramping, but it will have affects on any smooth muscle of the body. A great addition to any reproductive blend.

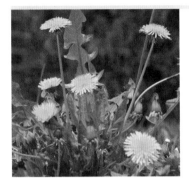

### DANDELION

*Taraxacum officinale*

PARTS USED leaves and roots    HELPFUL FOR day-to-day health, women's health, men's health, babies and children

Both the leaf and root of dandelion offer wonderful medicine that can easily be incorporated into your daily diet. The leaves are only slightly bitter, and the root makes any stir fry a bit more lively. The root is considered an alterative herb, meaning it helps optimize the nutrient uptake and waste output of the body and aids metabolism. This translates into helping the body clear toxins, so dandelion is often referred to as a blood cleanser. The leaves are diuretic and help the body maintain a healthy water balance. There have been reports of dandelion successfully reducing rheumatism, perhaps due to its ability to clear the body of built-up waste by-products.

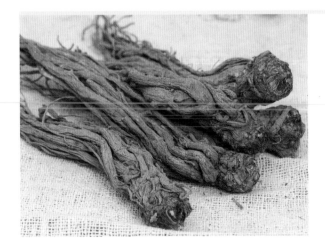

### DONG QUAI

*Angelica sinensis*

PARTS USED root    HELPFUL FOR women's health

Dong quai is a wonderful blood builder and blood mover often recommended for those who have pelvic stagnation, which leads to low menstrual flow or increased pain with menstruation. It is also a liver-supporting herb, so if you are inclined to believe the liver is involved in hormone imbalance, dong quai should be considered. You can make it into a tea or eat small amounts of the raw root each day. One of my teachers said to eat as much as the size of my pinky fingernail each day.

## ECHINACEA

*Echinacea purpurea*

PARTS USED roots    HELPFUL FOR day-to-day
health, immune defense, women's health,
babies and children, travel health

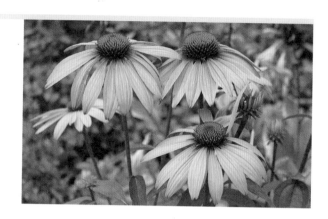

Everyone's favorite cold herb, echinacea is often misun-
derstood. Echinacea was one of the first herbs to hit the
mainstream market, and the research had yet to catch up.
Research shows that upon first use, echinacea activates
the white blood cells to increase and mobilize. This in
turn stimulates the immune system, causing the natural
defense cells to be on the lookout for foreign invaders.
Taking echinacea continuously does not produce a continuous spike in natural
defense; it is more a use-as-needed herb. If you are sitting next to a co-worker
who just went down with the flu, that is the time to take echinacea. You take it
in small doses several times a day the first day or two of a cold or illness to boost
your immune system's fighting powers, not continuously in hopes of building a
stronger immune system. If you are unable to ward off a cold or flu after 2 days
of taking echinacea, you must reexamine where the cold has settled and reassess
your herbal treatment going forward to minimize the duration of the illness.

Echinacea can be used for so much more than just stimulating the immune
response. Use it topically for skin infections or internally for digestive bacterial
infections. Some research shows that *Echinacea angustifolia* is helpful for cervical
dysplasia, and I often add echinacea to my pretravel tonics to protect me from
the varying bacteria experienced on travel days. For babies and children, using a
glycerin drop formula makes it easy to dispense, and the sweetness of the glycerin
typically makes it widely accepted.

## ELDERBERRY

*Sambucus nigra*

PARTS USED berries, flowers, and leaves    HELPFUL FOR day-
to-day health, immune defense, babies and children

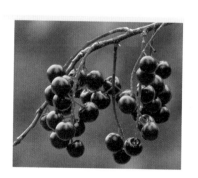

This plant with the little dark purple berry and the white elderflowers has really
made the scene over the last few years. Elderberry syrup is a common recom-
mendation for colds and flus, and it is said to be antiviral. Like most berries,
elderberries are high in bioflavinoids and have antioxidant properties, helping to

protect the body against free radicals and oxidative stress. An excellent research paper on elderberry created by the European Medicines Agency (Committee on Herbal Medicinal Products, "Assessment report on *Sambucus nigra* L., fructus," EMA/HMPC/44208/2012) demonstrates elderberry's effectiveness in relieving symptoms of influenza. I harvest it every year in the fall and make a big batch of elderberry syrup, often adding splashes to all of our water bottles. I often add varying ingredients to my syrups such as echinacea root, reishi mushroom, cinnamon, cloves—really whatever I have in the medicine cabinet that may help in time of need for a cold or flu.

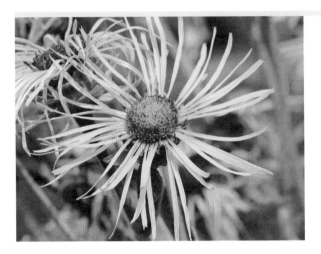

### ELECAMPANE

*Inula helenium*

PARTS USED roots    HELPFUL FOR immune defense, babies and children

I first learned about elecampane from my mentor, Linda Quintana of Wonderland Teas and Spices in Bellingham, Washington. She taught me of its incredible healing potential for the lungs and often recommended it for lung rehabilitation. I use it when colds last too long and get into the deeper recesses of the bronchial tubes. It helps to pull phlegm up and out of the respiratory tract and also works to heal damaged lung tissue.

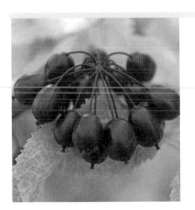

### ELEUTHERO

*Eleutherococcus senticosus*

PARTS USED roots    HELPFUL FOR day-to-day health, immune defense, women's health, men's health, emotional support, elders' health

There are many ginseng-type herbs, and eleuthero is one of them. Eleuthero is known as Siberian ginseng, distinguishing it from Chinese ginseng and American ginseng. It is neutral when it comes to temperature, meaning it doesn't have the same heat-producing effects as these other ginsengs. Eleuthero is also much less stimulating and much more nourishing than the others. It is a tonic herb, used to balance immunity, mood, hormones, and stress.

MUST-HAVE HERBS FOR DAY-TO-DAY USE

## EPIMEDIUM

*Epimedium sagittatum*

PARTS USED leaves    HELPFUL FOR men's health

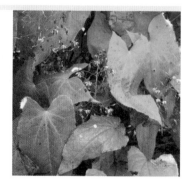

This herb is also known as horny goat weed because after several goats were seen eating it, their libidos seemed to increase. Now, I raised goats, and I'm not sure an increase in libido is possible with male goats, but we'll go with it. The active ingredient, icariin, has been shown to raise testosterone, and the herb overall has been shown to improve the circulation of testosterone and corticosterone and to raise nitric oxide levels in the body.

## FENNEL

*Foeniculum vulgare*

PARTS USED seeds    HELPFUL FOR day-to-day health, women's health, babies and children

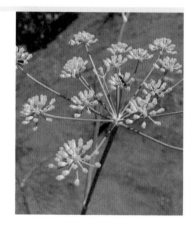

Great for stomach upset, cramping, and lower bowel complaints. When a stomachache is obviously due to overeating, constipation, or illness, fennel can quickly provide relief from gas, colic, and intestinal tension. Fennel helps to loosen phlegm and congestion, making coughs more productive, and helps relieve the dry, hacking cough of bronchitis. It is used in many recipes to increase lactation. A decoction of the seeds has traditionally been used for generalized eye irritation.

## GENTIAN

*Gentiana lutea*

PARTS USED roots    HELPFUL FOR day-to-day health, women's health, men's health

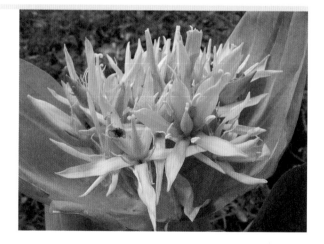

Digestive complaints often stem from what is eaten, stress, lack of proper digestive enzymes, medications, or eating too fast. The use of bitters—herbs that have a predominantly bitter taste, like gentian—is extremely helpful for almost any digestive complaint. Using bitters before a meal or at the onset of eating should help generate stomach acid to aid in the initial digestive process and support it through completion.

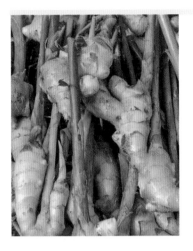

### GINGER

*Zingiber officinale*

PARTS USED roots    HELPFUL FOR day-to-day health, immune defense, women's health, babies and children, emotional support, travel health, elders' health

The anti-nausea herb, ginger is great for calming the stomach and relieving the sense of needing to vomit. This warming herb can be used throughout the body to reduce pain and cramping of the muscular kind. I recommend it when someone is experiencing a cold or flu but just can't quite mount the fever and immune response to kick it. Ginger will gently raise the fever to aid in burning out the infection invading the body. Ginger is also considered helpful to warm up the respiratory tract and release tension that may be restricting the ability to expel mucus.

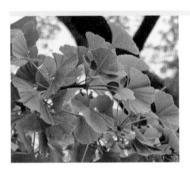

### GINKGO

*Ginkgo biloba*

PARTS USED leaf    HELPFUL FOR day-to-day health, men's health, emotional support, elders' health

Ginkgo is commonly known for its memory-boosting powers. It increases oxygenation to the brain, allowing for clearer thinking. This action doesn't affect just the brain, though. It can help reduce PMS, increase libido, and decrease anxiety and depression, and it has even been reported to reduce headaches and migraines.

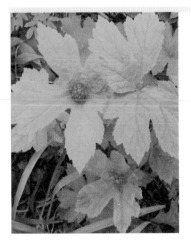

### GOLDENSEAL

*Hydrastis canadensis*

PARTS USED roots    HELPFUL FOR day-to-day health, immune defense, women's health, babies and children, travel health

This amazing herb is unfortunately no longer abundant in the wild due to over-harvesting, and because cultivating it is challenging, this herb has become very expensive. The double downside to this is that goldenseal's healing properties are hard to find in other herbs. Yes, other herbs contain berberine, which fights infection, but goldenseal's ability both to fight infection and to heal mucous membranes is an incredible combination. I use it internally and topically for various infections, and it is my go-to remedy for infections of the stomach and intestinal tract.

## HAWTHORN

*Crataegus laevigata*

PARTS USED berries, leaves, flowers   HELPFUL FOR day-to-day health, men's health, babies and children, emotional support, elders' health

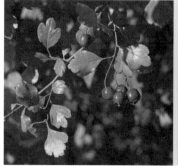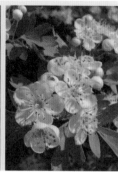

The berries, leaves, and flowers of hawthorn are all used in herbal medicine. The berries are specific to supporting the heart and cardiac function, whereas the leaves and flowers help circulation.

## HOPS

*Humulus lupulus*

PARTS USED strobiles (flowers)   HELPFUL FOR day-to-day health, immune defense, women's health, men's health, emotional support

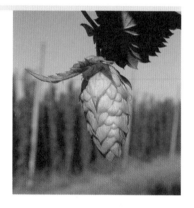

The flowers of the hop plant are called strobiles, and they have strong sedative effects. Working on both the nerves and the muscles, hops are helpful for many restless sleepers. Hops are bitter by nature and therefore work on the digestive system to varying degrees. I include hops in formulas for anxiety, sleep, digestive upset, and lactation. I find a little bit for the new mother helps her to relax into milk letdown and eases concerns over her ability to provide for her baby.

## HYSSOP

*Hyssopus officinalis*

PARTS USED leaves   HELPFUL FOR immune defense, babies and children

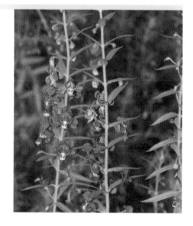

Sipped as a tea or taken as a tincture, hyssop has flu-fighting power, helping to ease muscle aches and respiratory congestion. It is known to increase circulation, which naturally mobilizes the immune system while also fighting infection. A gentle diaphoretic, it can also help to open up the pores to induce sweating when fever is present.

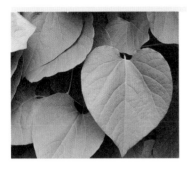

## KAVA KAVA

*Piper methysticum*

PARTS USED roots, rhizomes   HELPFUL FOR emotional support

A relatively new herb on the American market, kava has gained popularity as a sedative. It works by binding to various receptors in the brain, particularly the part of the brain known as the amygdala, which regulates feelings of fear and anxiety. It is also a muscle relaxant. Most people find deep relaxation in the use of kava.

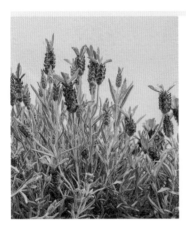

## LAVENDER

*Lavendula* species

PARTS USED flowers   HELPFUL FOR day-to-day complaints, immune defense, women's health, babies and children, emotional support, travel health, elders' health

Lavender flowers are pretty, and the volatile oils extracted from them offer a plethora of healing benefits. They are antimicrobial, antibacterial, sedative, carminative, and antispasmodic in nature. The oils are known to relieve tension, reduce headaches, soothe burns, expel gas, and calm upset stomachs and unsettled emotions. They are excellent for relieving heat and healing skin. Using lavender flowers is one of my favorite ways to introduce children to herbs. I often teach them how to create little lavender sachets, and it is rare to find a child who doesn't appreciate the smell. My daughter's preschool teacher would put a drop of lavendar oil on the children's palms for them to rub together and smell before nap time to calm the high energy of the classroom.

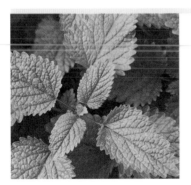

## LEMON BALM

*Melissa officinalis*

PARTS USED leaves   HELPFUL FOR day-to-day health, immune defense, women's health, babies and children, emotional support, travel health, elders' health

A gentle herb that calms overly excited nerves. Brew it up any time emotions have run high or stress is causing the heart to race or the stomach to churn. An antiviral, lemon balm has the ability to combat high viral loads. I often recommend it for dormant viral conditions such as shingles, herpes, and HPV. Its volatile oils also make it antimicrobial.

## LOBELIA

*Lobelia inflata*

PARTS USED leaves, flowers    HELPFUL FOR day-to-day health,
immune defense, men's health, elders' health

Lobelia is a field plant with emetic properties that if accidentally consumed
causes purging. There is a story about a young boy who liked to play tricks on
people and would give them lobelia. The odd thing was, while each person wasn't
too happy about the experience, they all reported feeling amazing afterward.
Lobelia has an incredible ability to purge the body, but it doesn't need to be in a
violent way. Typically we use it to support the respiratory tract by opening and
clearing the lungs. I've also used small amounts to increase sluggish circulation
in order to warm up cold hands and feet. It has a very relaxing effect, and some
use it to help induce sleep.

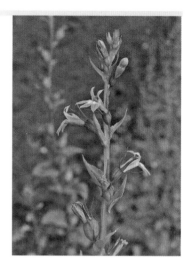

## MOTHERWORT

*Leonurus cardiaca*

PARTS USED leaves, stems, flowers    HELPFUL FOR women's health

One of my favorite herbs, this one grows tall and is considered one of the plants
to have outside your home to provide protection from negative energies. It has
been used as heart medicine for centuries. It can calm and nourish the heart,
and research shows it can decrease artery calcification. Motherwort also works
on the endocrine system in supporting hormone balance. New research shows
promising results from using it to treat Graves' disease.

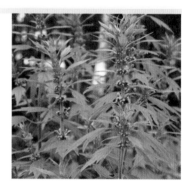

## MUGWORT

*Artemisia vulgaris*

PARTS USED leaves and stems    HELPFUL FOR
day-to-day health, women's health

A sedative and liver tonic, mugwort is most commonly known to
activate the dream cycles while we sleep. This is great if you are
trying to remember and process your dreams, but not so great if
you already have an active dream time, as it can leave one feeling
quite tired in the morning from too much stimulation. Its liver
actions help maintain hormone balance and seem to target the
problem of menstrual irregularity.

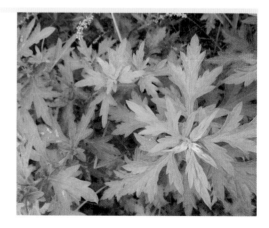

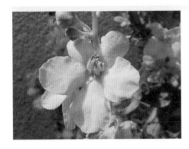

## MULLEIN

*Verbascum thapsus*

PARTS USED flowers and leaves  HELPFUL FOR day-to-day health, immune defense, babies and children

Mullein is a helpful herb to treat any cold. It moves mucus up and out while also calming respiratory irritation. The flowers of the mullein plant, which must be harvested and processed fresh, are an excellent tonic for ear pain and infection.

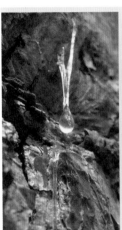
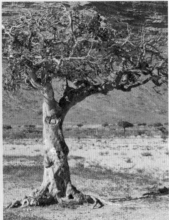

## MYRRH

*Commiphora myrrha*

PARTS USED oleo gum resin from the stem  HELPFUL FOR day-to-day health, immune defense, women's health, babies and children, travel health

Myrrh is a resin extracted from the bark of a small, thorny tree. Shown to have antibacterial, antifungal, anti-microbial, and antiseptic effects, myrrh is a great herb for colds and flus. I use it most for its drying capabilities, particularly for the drip-drip-drip of a runny nose. It can also open up nasal passageways, making sleep easier when there is congestion.

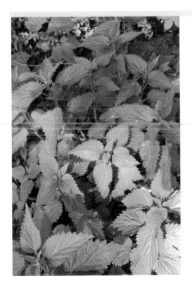

## NETTLE

*Urtica dioica*

PARTS USED leaves, roots, seeds  HELPFUL FOR day-to-day health, men's health, women's health

Nettle leaf, root, and seed are all used in herbal medicine and are anti-inflammatory. The seed is most commonly used in kidney blends, and both the leaf and root are used in prostate and male reproductive medicines. I've traditionally used nettle leaf anytime I've seen the need for a patient to get increased B vitamins and minerals. This can be due to generalize fatigued, laxity in ligaments, decreased breast milk, or debilitated functioning of one or more bodily systems. The leaves contain quercetin, which is helpful for seasonal allergy relief. Nettle leaf can also treat bladder weakness, and its astringency is called upon when it is used to treat excessive bleeding or leucorrhea. Also helpful in hair tonics.

## OATSTRAW

*Avena sativa*

PARTS USED stems and leaves   HELPFUL FOR day-to-day
health, babies and children, emotional support

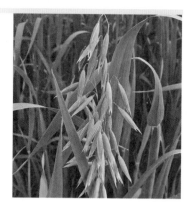

Oatstraw is one of those unassuming herbs that rarely gets talked about much anymore. Many people believe only the milky oat tops have medicinal value, but I prefer to use the oatstraw, believing it a better choice for long-term nourishing support. It is very gentle in action and packed with nutrients. This makes it helpful to anyone who has burned the candle at both ends and feels chronically run down and stressed.

## OREGON GRAPE

*Mahonia aquifolium*

PARTS USED rhizomes, roots   HELPFUL FOR day-to-day health, immune
defense, women's health, babies and children, travel health

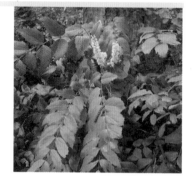

Oregon grape is an herb that works toward creating balance in the body. I've used it successfully for both diarrhea and constipation. It contains berberine, a powerful antibacterial agent. When something is off with the digestive system, I reach for Oregon grape first. It has traditionally been used for those who feel bloated, tired, toxic, and unconnected to their body.

## PARTRIDGE BERRY

*Mitchella repens*

PARTS USED berry   HELPFUL FOR day-
to-day health, women's health

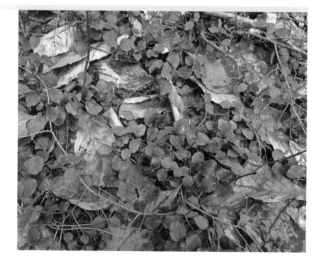

I find partridge berry a great herb for the overachieving woman—the woman who is stretched thin by all she has going on yet maintains it surprisingly well. Whether it shows or not, this does take a toll, and partridge berry does a great job of nourishing those who may be depleted. In combination it also calms and can be helpful for anxiety. A superior herb if dealing with infertility and menstrual irregularity, and very useful when bladder infections or inflammation arise.

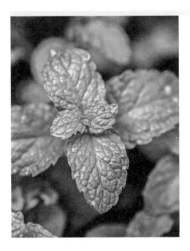

## PEPPERMINT

*Mentha ×piperita*

PARTS USED leaves   HELPFUL FOR day-to-day health, immune defense, women's health, men's health, babies and children, emotional support, travel health, elders' health

A simple stimulant that can soothe the stomach, open the respiratory tract, and calm the central nervous system. Drink peppermint leaf tea to quell nausea, decrease muscle aches, and relieve the head of congestion. My favorite head cold remedy is a cup of peppermint tea, as I can breathe in the volatile oils that roll off the steam while I'm drinking it. These volatile oils work quickly and effectively. A few drops of essential oil to the temples or the nape of the neck have proven effective to calm tension headaches.

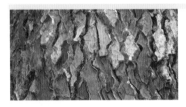

## PINE

*Pinus pinaster*

PARTS USED bark   HELPFUL FOR day-to-day health, men's health

Pine bark is most often used for erectile dysfunction, but I use it for high cholesterol and to address sluggish circulation.

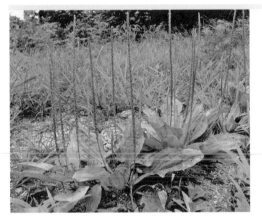

## PLANTAIN

*Plantago major*

PARTS USED leaves, roots, seeds   HELPFUL FOR day-to-day health, women's health, babies and children, travel health

Plantain leaf is one of the herbs I consider a panacea. When in doubt, I try plantain. It soothes irritation, calms inflammation, draws out pain and infection, and heals mucous membranes and skin. It has also traditionally been used to soothe ulcers and toothaches, ease hoarseness of the voice, and rid the body of excess mucus. Teaching your child how to identify plantain at an early age will provide her or him with a lifetime of yellow jacket sting relief. Stings hurt, and the quicker you can put something helpful on them, the better. Finding a few leaves, chewing them up, and spitting them onto the sting is not only super fun for kids, it also distracts them and makes them proactive in helping themselves. The best part? It relieves the pain.

## RASPBERRY

*Rubus idaeus*

PARTS USED leaves    HELPFUL FOR day-to-day health, women's health, men's health, babies and children, elders' health, travel health

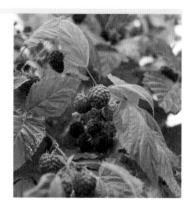

In women's health, raspberry (also commonly called red raspberry) is most often considered a nourishing tonic during pregnancy to prepare the uterus for delivery. Raspberry is also a superior gastrointestinal herb and used often for diarrhea and irritable bowel syndrome. Its astringent nature and high nutrient content make it very supportive to the physical body. It aids in fever management, and I often add it to my cold and flu teas due to its high vitamin C content.

## RHODIOLA

*Rhodiola rosea*

PARTS USED root bark    HELPFUL FOR emotional support

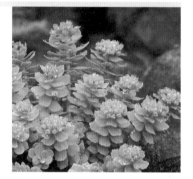

This is one of two adaptogen herbs (schisandra is the other) that are superior at supporting the adrenal glands and regulating the cortisol stress response. Both work to balance the function of the adrenals and return the body to normal cortisol release when someone has been living in a constant stress response cycle. When a patient reports chronic stress with symptoms of anxiety or insomnia, I typically include one of these herbs to provide support.

## ROSE

*Rosa* species

PARTS USED petals, hips    HELPFUL FOR day-to-day health, immune defense

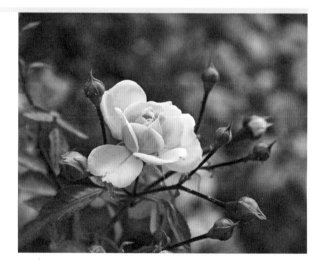

Roses seem to radiate peace. Just looking at one can evoke a sense of calm in my body, and the scent has an intoxicating effect upon my brain. While using roses in this way provides emotional healing, using them internally helps to stop bleeding. Rose petals were traditionally used for internal pains of the body, including headaches, tooth pain, sore throat, and stomach upset; for irritations of the respiratory tract; and for chronic, unproductive coughs.

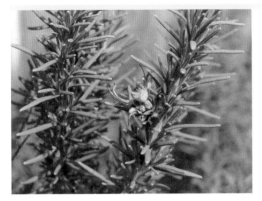

## ROSEMARY

*Rosmarinus officinalis*

PARTS USED leaves    HELPFUL FOR day-to-day health, immune defense, women's health, babies and children, elders' health

A stimulating herb, rosemary wakes us up and gets the brain juices flowing. It is often included in memory blends to stimulate cognitive function. I also add it in smaller quantities to dream blends to help people remember their dreams. Rosemary can be used to treat respiratory infections that present with excessive mucus and a wet cough. Its stimulating nature can also warm the skin and extremities by moving the blood. It was traditionally used to raise low blood pressure and stimulate circulation, so use it with caution if you are on medications for such conditions. High in volatile oils, rosemary is an herb to plant along the pathway to your front door to purify guests before they enter.

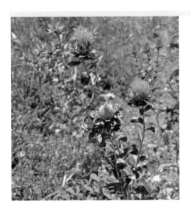

## SAFFLOWER

*Carthamus tinctorius*

PARTS USED flower    HELPFUL FOR immune support, women's health, men's health

Although it does have blood-thinning properties, the delicate safflower is in my opinion an extremely underutilized herb. It has a tendency to travel to small spaces in the body, and it is exactly these small spaces where waste can accumulate. Safflower gently pushes out toxic build-up and decreases the potential for long-term damage to such areas as the joints and arteries. It is supportive in lowering cholesterol and blood pressure, and I use it to prevent blood clots.

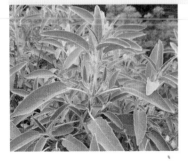

## SAGE

*Salvia officinalis*

PARTS USED leaves    HELPFUL FOR day-to-day health, immune defense, women's health, babies and children

Almost any sore throat will benefit from sage leaf tea. Its soothing effects work to calm inflammation, and it is antibacterial and antiseptic. Drink it for systemic effects and gargle for target treatment to the throat. A great addition to any cold tea blend, it will work to break up congestion and relieve the discomforts of colds.

## SAW PALMETTO

*Serenoa repens*

PARTS USED berries HELPFUL FOR men's health

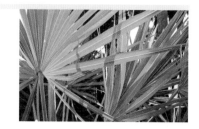

Saw palmetto is the most commonly prescribed herb for male prostate problems. It works to balance hormones of the reproductive system and seems to normalize the functioning of the prostate.

## SCHISANDRA

*Schisandra chinensis*

PARTS USED berries HELPFUL FOR day-to-day health, women's health, emotional support

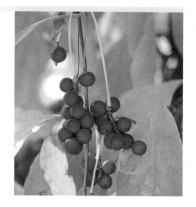

This is one of two adaptogen herbs (rhodiola is the other) that are superior at supporting the adrenal glands and regulating the cortisol stress response. Both work to balance the function of the adrenals and return the body to normal cortisol release when someone has been living in a constant stress response cycle. When a patient reports chronic stress with symptoms of anxiety or insomnia, I typically include one of these herbs to provide support.

## SILK TASSEL

*Garrya eliptica*

PARTS USED leaf HELPFUL FOR women's health

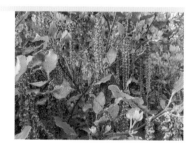

Another wonderful herb that comes to the rescue when menstrual cramping is on the rise, silk tassel is a strong antispamodic. If you are experiencing gastrointestinal cramping with bowel upset, silk tassel will work wonders in relieving you of the discomforts. It is extremely bitter and can be used as a quinine substitute.

## SKULLCAP

*Scutellaria lateriflora*

PARTS USED leaves HELPFUL FOR day-to-day health, women's health, emotional support

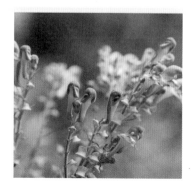

A superior nutritive nervine that works to calm the nerves and give resilience. When we do too much in our lives, we tend to become depleted, and our stress centers become overactive. This can lead to excessive thinking and an inability to calm ourselves. Skullcap works to quiet the mind and clarify thoughts. Skullcap is also helpful to treat pain that inhibits sleep and for insomnia itself.

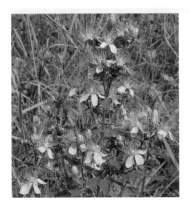

## ST. JOHN'S WORT

*Hypericum perforatum*

PARTS USED leaves, flowers    HELPFUL FOR day-to-day health,
immune support, women's health, emotional support

St. John's wort got its name from its traditional flowering and harvesting day—
St. John's Day, June 24. Traditionally used for nerve pain and irritation, St. John's
wort is an herb I've given to those suffering from neuralgia, neuropathy, and
exposed nerve sensitivities. These days the research on St. John's wort is focused
on its antidepressent effects, and I often add it to tea blends for this purpose. My
patients like the subtle effect it seems to create, gently lifting the mood.

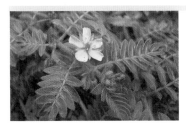

## TRIBULUS

*Tribulus terrestris*

PARTS USED fruit    HELPFUL FOR men's health

Also known as puncturevine, this low-growing plant with a prickly-looking
thorn has been proven to raise testosterone levels. This improves libido and
stamina, and many men report an increase in their sense of vitality.

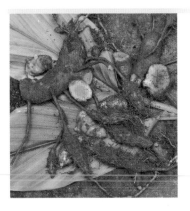

## TURMERIC

*Curcuma longa*

PARTS USED roots    HELPFUL FOR day-to-day health, immune
defense, women's health, men's health, elders' health

More and more research is coming out regarding the anti-inflammatory properties of turmeric. By adding turmeric to your diet, you can make your food
into powerful medicine. Used for arthritis, rheumatism, and aches and pains,
turmeric has the ability to move the blood and warm the tissues. Considered
a blood purifier, turmeric can remove toxins from the blood and reduce the
accumulation of metabolic by-products.

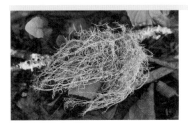

## USNEA

*Usnea barbata*

PARTS USED whole plant    HELPFUL FOR day-to-day health,
immune defense, women's health, travel health

Usnea is a type of lichen that can be seen throughout the forests of the Pacific
Northwest, looking like witches' hair falling from the tree branches. Several lichens

MUST-HAVE HERBS FOR DAY-TO-DAY USE

look similar, and proper identification is important. Usnea is a must-have for the immune defense medicine cabinet. Stephen Buhner's book *Herbal Antibiotics* discusses its antibiotic properties, and I often use it when I suspect a bacterial infection such as strep throat or when the flu comes on quickly with a high fever. Usnea needs to be cut up finely with scissors before being used in teas and tinctures.

## VERVAIN

*Verbena officinalis*

PARTS USED leaf   HELPFUL FOR day-to-day health

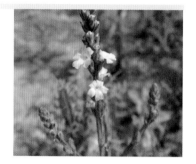

When anxious feelings pervade, particularly when one questions one's worth, I reach for vervain, a true nervine. It is calming and works as a tonic to both the central nervous and reproductive systems. Vervain can increase breast milk and quell dysmenorrhea when taken as a long-term tonic. Vervain may be the right choice for tension or menstrual headache relief as well.

## VITEX

*Vitex agnus-castus*

PARTS USED seed, berries   HELPFUL FOR women's health

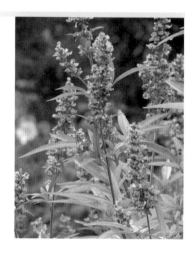

In ancient Greece, this herb was associated with chastity. Given to all of the maidens before marriage rites, it was also considered a fertility booster. It is an adaptogen by nature, meaning it helps to create balance—whatever is low it raises, and whatever is high it lowers. Typically estrogen is dominant, so vitex works to lower it and to raise progesterone. This herb is often used for absence of menses, irregular menses, and other hormonal troubles such as acne, but it requires patience and consistent dosing. Those with polycystic ovary syndrome (PCOS) need to consult with their natural health care provider before using vitex, as not all PCOS patients will benefit from the herb.

## WILD YAM

*Dioscorea villosa*

PARTS USED root   HELPFUL FOR women's health

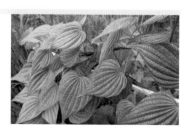

A root with estrogen-driving properties, wild yam is helpful when you are experiencing hormonal imbalance and it is causing vaginal dryness, PMS, bone loss, and/or decreased libido. Wild yam also has powerful antispasmodic and anti-inflammatory properties. A good herb to consider when joint pain is present or if gastrointestinal cramping is causing discomfort.

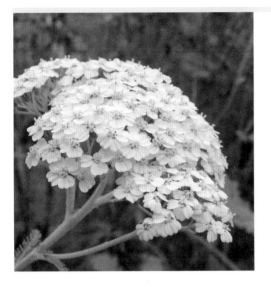

## YARROW

*Achillea millefolium*

PARTS USED flowers, leaves, stems  HELPFUL FOR day-to-day health, immune defense, women's health, babies and children, emotional support, travel health

Yarrow is a gentle fever reducer and a powerful hemostatic. It is readily used for many different skin conditions, including bruising, wounds, bleeding, and pain; and for hot, stagnant conditions where blood is not moving well, including in the digestive tract, the circulatory system, and the reproductive system. When a cold and or fever strikes my kids and they are obviously ill (wanting to lie down), a small cup or even a few teaspoons of yarrow tea can alleviate the discomforts of fever, promote gentle sweating, stimulate the immune system, and improve the mood.

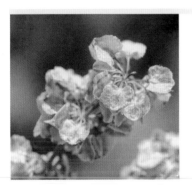

## YELLOW DOCK

*Rumex crispus*

PARTS USED roots  HELPFUL FOR day-to-day health, women's health, elders' health

This herb is helpful for hormone regulation through supporting the liver and is often recommended when assimilation of iron is a problem. It is often used in women's reproductive formulas. Yellow dock was traditionally used to treat swollen, painful, and itchy skin. It is also helpful for lower digestive complaints where food feels like it isn't going anywhere.

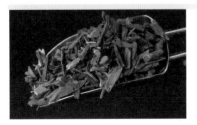

## YOHIMBE

*Pausinystalia johimbe*

PARTS USED bark  HELPFUL FOR men's health

Yohimbe contains a chemical called yohimbine that can increase blood flow and nerve impulses to the penis. It is most commonly used as needed to treat erectile dysfunction and decreased libido.

# Day-to-Day Health

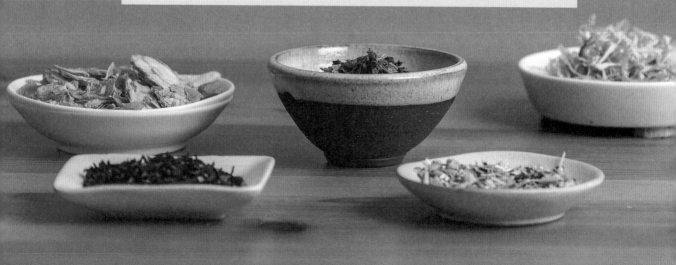

"To experience peace does not mean that your life is always blissful. It means that you are capable of tapping into a blissful state of mind amidst the normal chaos of a hectic life."

JILL BOLTE TAYLOR

CARING FOR ONESELF is rarely taught in our culture, but it is necessary. In this section you'll find recipes to address almost every day-to-day health challenge you might encounter. Again, these recipes are not to replace professional care if you encounter serious health concerns. These recipes are to reunite you with the knowledge of how to care for yourself for the minor complaints that humans sometimes deal with. Having the ability to care for yourself and your family by treating such common conditions as colds, stomachaches, and headaches is empowering. I hope the recipes in this chapter will help you to reclaim the confidence to give your body what it needs during times of discomfort. Remember, unless noted, dried herbs should be used in the recipes.

## ≡ ACNE ≡

Whether you are a teenager or an adult, acne can cause upset. Not only is it an ego bruise, but it can be quite painful as well. Try the recipes here to prevent, minimize, or treat problem areas.

## Acne-Fighting Face Scrub

*Use this for a case of noninflammatory acne.*

1 tablespoon rose petals

1 tablespoon chickweed leaf

1 tablespoon uncooked oatmeal,
   gluten free if necessary

1 tablespoon honey

$1/8$ cup olive oil

In an herb grinder, slightly grind rose petals, chickweed leaves, and oatmeal. Do not grind into a powder. Transfer to a clean bowl and add the honey and olive oil. Mix together well. Wash your face with your normal cleanser and then apply the scrub with your fingertips. Massaging the scrub in small circles, gently move around your face for 1 or 2 minutes and then rinse with warm water. For a deeper moisturizing effect, leave on your face for 5 minutes. End by splashing cool water onto your face and dry.

# Blackheads-B-Gone Mask

1 tablespoon plantain leaf powder

1 tablespoon chamomile flower powder

1 tablespoon comfrey leaf powder

1 tablespoon bentonite clay powder

Mix all the powders together in a clean bowl. Add a touch of hot water and mix into a paste. You need enough water to get a smooth application. With too little water, the mask will not stay in place on your face. Once the desired consistency has been reached, apply to your face evenly. Avoid the eye area. Leave on your face for 10 to 15 minutes and then rinse with warm water.

# Breakout-Prevention Spray

2 tablespoons burdock root

1 tablespoon calendula flower

2 tablespoons wild lettuce leaf

1 teaspoon black walnut hull

witch hazel extract

20 drops clary sage essential oil

Place the herbs in a glass mason jar and cover completely with the witch hazel extract to a depth of at least 1 or 2 inches. Once the herbs have become saturated, add a little more witch hazel if needed to cover. Cap tightly and put in a cool, dark place like a cupboard or pantry for 2 weeks, shaking every day. Strain and transfer to a spray bottle. Add the essential oil and shake well. Every day after cleansing your face, spray onto your face and use a cotton pad to wipe away gently.

# Skin-Clearing Toner Spray

*Use this for cystic (inflammatory) acne.*

2 tablespoons wild lettuce leaf

2 tablespoons plantain leaf

1 tablespoon black walnut hull

1 teaspoon chaparral leaf

witch hazel extract

20 drops juniper essential oil

Place the herbs in a glass mason jar and cover completely with the witch hazel extract to a depth of at least 1 or 2 inches. Once the herbs have become saturated, add a little more witch hazel if needed to cover. Cap tightly and put in a cool, dark place like a cupboard or pantry for 2 weeks, shaking every day. Strain and transfer to a spray bottle. Add the essential oil and shake well. Every day after cleansing your face, spray onto your face and use a cotton pad to wipe away gently.

# Cystic Blaster Formula with Variations

*If painful pustules are a part of your regular day to day, try this blend to clear the system of possible causes such as inflammation, hormone imbalance, metabolic by-products, or stress.*

### TEA VARIATION

1 ounce dandelion root

1 ounce yellow dock root

1 ounce echinacea root

½ ounce Oregon grape root

½ ounce skullcap leaf

Mix the herbs in a bowl and store in a glass jar. Use 4 to 5 tablespoons to make 1-quart batches. Drink 2 to 3 cups per day for 6 to 8 weeks, or as needed.

### CAPSULE VARIATION

Halve the receipe above, using the herbs in powder form, and mix the powders in a bowl. Fill 200 empty capsules. Take 2 capsules twice per day.

### TINCTURE VARIATION

1 teaspoon dandelion root

1 teaspoon yellow dock root

1 teaspoon echinacea root

½ teaspoon Oregon grape root

½ teaspoon skullcap leaf

2 ounces vodka

Put all herbs in a 2-ounce glass jar. Cover with vodka, close, and shake well. Put in a cool, dark place like a cupboard or pantry for 3 weeks, shaking every day. Strain and transfer to a dropper bottle. Take 2 dropperfuls twice daily.

# Acne Spot Treatment

*Use this to treat breakouts and painful nodules.*

plantain leaf powder

chickweed leaf powder

If you can't obtain plantain leaf and chickweed leaf powdered, you can purchase dried leaves (or pick them fresh from your backyard and allow to dry) and grind in your herb grinder. Mix equal parts of these two herbs and keep in a jar. When needed, put a small amount in a bowl and add just enough hot water to make a paste. Let cool slightly and then apply to affected areas. Leave on for 20 minutes. For an extra boost, apply a warm compress over the application. This can be done by having a bowl of hot water and a small washcloth close by that you can soak in the water and wring out.

# ⟨ ACNE ROSACEA ⟩

Rosacea has been considered acne and an inflammatory process. However you wish to classify it, its presentation is consistent: a redness that spreads over the cheeks and nose. It often presents as small bumps that may or may not have pus in them, and the capillaries of the face are affected. Sometimes it is chronic and other times it comes on with certain stressors: food, emotional upset, environmental toxins. Use the following two recipes for prevention and treatment.

## Rosacea-Erasing Tea

1 ounce burdock root

½ ounce feverfew leaf

½ ounce yarrow flower

½ ounce licorice root

¼ ounce gentian root

1 ounce peppermint leaf

Mix the herbs in a bowl and store in a glass jar. Use 4 to 5 tablespoons to make 1-quart batches. Drink 2 to 3 cups per day for 6 to 8 weeks, or as needed.

## Rosacea-Erasing Capsules

½ ounce burdock root powder

½ ounce peppermint leaf powder

¼ ounce feverfew leaf powder

¼ ounce yarrow flower powder

¼ ounce licorice root powder

¼ ounce gentian root powder

Mix the powders in a bowl and fill 200 empty capsules. Take 2 capsules twice per day.

# ⟹ ALLERGIES ⟸

See also "Hay Fever." The key to allergy relief is to decrease histamine release and soothe mucous membranes, which aids in relieving symptoms.

## Allergy-Tamer Capsules

½ ounce nettle leaf powder

½ ounce calendula flower powder

½ ounce fennel seed powder

½ ounce yerba santa leaf powder

Mix the powders in a bowl and fill 200 empty capsules. Take 2 capsules twice per day.

## Allergy-Tamer Tea

1½ ounces rose hips

1 ounce yerba santa leaf

½ ounce nettle leaf

½ ounce orange peel

½ ounce lemongrass

Mix the herbs in a bowl and store in a glass jar. Use 4 to 5 tablespoons to make 1-quart batches. Drink 2 to 3 cups per day for 6 to 8 weeks, or as needed.

## NETI POT FORMULA FOR ALLERGIES

When you experience allergies, it is very important to care for your respiratory system and the mucous membranes that are under attack. One of the best ways to do this is to use a neti pot twice a day. I can attest to their positive results in clearing out particles that have been inhaled that are causing problems. By rinsing these from your nasal system, you are decreasing the overall irritant load. Try adding 1 dropper of wild cherry bark tincture to your neti pot along with the usual salt (follow the instructions that come with the pot). Wild cherry bark is known to help decrease histamine reactions in the body.

There are two types of anemia: iron deficiency and what is called pernicious anemia, which is a deficiency of the vitamin B12.

## Iron-Boosting Syrup

1 ounce yellow dock root

1 ounce fenugreek seed

½ ounce anise seed

½ ounce nettle leaf

½ ounce dandelion leaf

¼ ounce cinnamon chips

8 cups water

2 cups blackstrap molasses

1 cup honey

Put the herbs in a saucepan with the water. Bring to a boil and simmer over medium-low heat until reduced by half. Strain out the herbs and put the brew back in the pan. Add blackstrap molasses and honey and gently heat to mix if necessary. Store in an amber bottle. Take 1 tablespoon daily.

## B12-Boosting Tea

1 ounce nettle leaf

1½ ounces hawthorn berry

½ ounce alfalfa leaf

½ ounce eleuthero root

½ ounce licorice root

Mix the herbs in a bowl and store in a glass jar. Use 4 to 5 tablespoons to make 1-quart batches. Drink 2 to 3 cups per day for 6 to 8 weeks, or as needed.

# ≡ APPETITE, DECREASED ≡

While our nation is obsessed with weight loss, many people suffer from decreased appetite. It is truly a struggle to never have a craving for food or the desire to eat.

## Appetite-Stimulating Bitters

*Bitters are a great way to stimulate the digestive juices and increase potential appetite.*

1 ounce gentian root

1 ounce yellow dock root

1 ounce fennel seed

1 ounce ginger root

8 ounces apple cider vinegar

Put all herbs into an 8-ounce glass jar and fill to the top with apple cider vinegar. Close tightly and shake well. Keep in a cupboard or pantry for 2 weeks, shaking the jar daily. Strain and transfer to a dropper bottle. Take 2 dropperfuls 15 minutes before a meal.

## Appetite-Building Teas

*These teas will help you build up a regular appetite. The first variation, using simply agrimony or wormwood leaf, addresses the upper or lower end of the digestive system that can be causing the decreased appetite. The second and third variations have a bit more flavor and add digestive bitters.*

### VARIATION 1

1 teaspoon agrimony leaf or

  1 teaspoon wormwood leaf

Steep 10 minutes in 10 ounces of hot water, covered. Drink 1 hour before mealtime.

### VARIATION 2

1 ounce agrimony leaf

½ ounce angelica root

½ ounce mugwort leaf

2 ounces peppermint leaf

Mix the herbs in a bowl and store in a glass jar. Steep 1 or 2 teaspoons in 10 ounces of hot water, covered, for 10 minutes, and drink 1 hour before mealtime.

## VARIATION 3

1 ounce centaury leaf

1 ounce blessed thistle leaf

¾ ounce gentian root

½ ounce ginger root

¾ ounce lemongrass

Mix the herbs in a bowl and store in a glass jar. Steep 1 or 2 teaspoons in 10 ounces of hot water, covered, for 10 minutes, and drink 1 hour before mealtime.

# ≡ ASTHMA ≡

The inability to breathe is a scary and life-threatening situation. These formulas are by no means an attempt to replace medications necessary to control asthma, but my experience has shown that they can lead to a decrease in the frequency and quantity of medications required.

## Better-Breathing Tincture

1½ ounces yerba santa leaf

1¼ ounces black cohosh root

1 ounce cramp bark

¼ ounce lobelia leaf

$\frac{1}{16}$ ounce cayenne powder

4 ounces vodka

Place all the herbs in a 4-ounce glass jar. Cover with vodka to a depth of 1 to 2 inches. Close and shake well. Put in a cool, dark place like a cupboard or pantry for 3 weeks, shaking every day. Strain and transfer to a dropper bottle. Take 2 dropperfuls twice daily or as needed, not to exceed six doses per day.

# DR. CHRISTOPHER'S LOBELIA TREATMENT

Many years ago I read a testimony from herbal master Dr. John Christopher regarding the use of lobelia for asthma. It inspired me, and after speaking with a patient, we decided to give it a go and had some success with it. Lobelia is emetic by nature, known as a strong cleansing agent that often leaves the patient feeling stronger and more vital after the purge. With asthma, an excessive amount of mucus sits consistently in the lungs. This treatment seems to pull out the mucus, clearing the lungs for perhaps the first time. Please do not consider doing this treatment without practitioner guidance, preferably from a trained herbalist or naturopathic physician who specializes in herbs.

1 cup peppermint tea
30 minutes later, 2 dropperfuls of lobelia tincture
15 minutes later, 2 more dropperfuls of lobelia tincture

Typically soon thereafter is a vomiting session. Rest afterward as needed.

## ATHLETE'S FOOT

Athlete's foot is a contagious fungal infection that often leads to a red scaly rash that itches.

## Antifungal Powder

2 ounces bentonite clay
1 ounce chaparral powder

1 ounce black walnut hull powder

Combine all the powders and put into a shaker bottle. Use twice daily after showers and in shoes to reduce the infection.

# Antifungal Tea

*Treating from the inside out while also treating the exterior surface is extremely helpful when it comes to fungal infections.*

1¼ ounces pau d'arco bark

1 ounce yarrow flower

1 ounce goldenseal root

½ ounce lavender flower

¼ ounce whole cloves

Mix the herbs in a bowl and store in a glass jar. Use 4 to 5 tablespoons to make 1-quart batches. Drink 2 to 3 cups per day for 6 to 8 weeks, or as needed.

# Antifungal Oil

*Rubbing an antifungal oil into your feet or wherever the fungus is can target treatment effectively. The key is using a light oil that is readily absorbed. In this recipe I recommend apricot oil.*

½ ounce wormwood leaf

¼ ounce usnea

½ ounce yarrow flower

½ ounce chaparral leaf

½ ounce black walnut hull

8–12 ounces apricot oil

40 drops tea tree essential oil

Grind all the herbs down from their whole dried form. It doesn't need to be a powder, just broken down a bit. Usnea can be tough, so use scissors to cut it up if needed. Another option is to put all the herbs into a blender, add the oil, and blend a bit before putting into the oven. Put the herbs in a glass baking dish and pour in enough oil to cover them 1 or 2 inches deep. Bake in the oven at 170 degrees F for 4 hours. Strain and transfer the oil to container of your choice. Add the essential oil. Rub 1 teaspoon into the affected area on each foot twice daily.

# ≡ BAD BREATH ≡

Poor oral hygiene as well as stomach issues can lead to chronic bad breath. It's best to investigate by visiting the dentist or your family practitioner if it persists.

## Mint Spirits Spray

½ ounce peppermint leaf

½ ounce spearmint leaf

¼ ounce anise seed

vegetable glycerin

40 drops peppermint essential oil

Put the herbs into a jar and cover them completely with vegetable glycerin to a depth of 1 or 2 inches. Close tightly and store in a cupboard or pantry for 3 weeks, shaking every day. Strain and add the essential oil. Shake well to mix and store in a spray bottle. Spray 1 to 3 sprays into the mouth when desired.

## Mouth Rinse

1 teaspoon caraway seed

2 teaspoons anise seed

1 teaspoon sage leaf

8 ounces hot water

Let the herbs steep in the hot water, covered, for 1 hour. Strain and transfer the infusion into a clean bottle. Gargle 1 to 2 ounces 3 times a day and spit out afterward.

## Stomach-Balancing Tea

*The focus of this tea is to correct any stomach imbalance that may be causing the halitosis.*

2 ounces chamomile flower

1 ounce marshmallow root

½ ounce dandelion leaf

½ ounce licorice root

Mix the herbs in a bowl and store in a glass jar. Make tea by the cup. Steep 1 or 2 teaspoons in 10 ounces of hot water, covered, for 10 minutes, and drink 1 cup twice daily between meals.

Bee stings, mosquito bites, and spider bites can all lead to painful inflammation and often an insatiable itch. Please keep in mind that most "bee" stings are actually yellow jacket stings. Honey and mason bees rarely sting unless provoked, whereas yellow jackets seem to like to actively get up into our human business.

## Fresh-Sting Poultice

2 plantain leaves                    1 sage leaf
A pinch of chickweed leaf

The herbalist way: stick all of these into your mouth and begin chewing. Chew it all up and mix it with your saliva. Then spit it out onto the sting for quick-acting relief.

The other way: put all the herbs in a mortar and use a pestle to grind them down. Transfer to a clean bowl and add a tiny bit of hot water to mix them together. (Don't add hot water to the herbs in your mortar. Most of them are made with porous material and the heat can cause the herbs to be drawn deep into the pores of the mortar.) Let cool slightly and place this herb cake on the sting.

## Drawing-Sting Paste

*The bromelain or papain found in meat tenderizer is extremely helpful to draw out the sting.*

1 ounce bentonite clay                    ½ ounce meat tenderizer
½ ounce plantain leaf powder

Mix all the ingredients and store in a glass jar. As needed, mix just enough powder and hot water together to make a paste, and apply to the affected area. Leave on for 30 minutes, applying 1 to 3 times per day.

# Bug Bite Itch-Relief Salve

1 tablespoon chaparral leaf

1 tablespoon white oak bark

1 tablespoon mugwort leaf

¾ cup olive oil

½ ounce beeswax

40–60 drops lavender essential oil

Put all the herbs into a glass baking dish and add enough olive oil to cover the herbs 1 or 2 inches deep. Bake in the oven at 170 degrees F for 4 hours and then strain. Put the strained oil in a saucepan and add the beeswax. Gently heat until the beeswax is melted, stirring continuously. Turn off the heat and pour into container of your choice. Add drops of lavender essential oil until the scent is as strong as you prefer. Apply as needed.

# Sting-Cooling Spray

1 tablespoon fresh arnica flowers

1 tablespoon fresh St. Johns' wort flowers

1 tablespoon fresh chickweed leaf

½ cup white vinegar

Submerge all the herbs in a jar with the vinegar. Close tightly and give it a good shake. Store in a cupboard or pantry for 3 weeks, shaking daily. Strain and transfer to a spray bottle. Spray 1 or 2 sprays onto affected areas.

## ≡ BLEEDING GUMS ≡

Bleeding gums can be caused by infection, improper hygiene, or improper care such as brushing too hard.

# Gum-Rinse Tincture

½ teaspoon goldenseal root

½ teaspoon white oak bark

½ teaspoon calendula flower

½ teaspoon myrrh resin

1 ounce vodka

Put the herbs in a 1-ounce jar and fill to the top with vodka. Close the jar tightly and shake well. Store in a cupboard or pantry for 14 days, shaking daily. Strain and put into a 1-ounce dropper bottle. Add 1 to 2 dropperfuls to 1 ounce of water and swish in mouth for 1 minute twice daily. Spit out afterward.

# ≡ BOILS ≡

A boil is an infection that begins in a hair follicle and the surrounding area. It is typically quite painful and often ends up filled with pus. The idea is to treat the infection, the inflammation, and the pain.

## Boil-Drawing Salve

1 tablespoon burdock root

1 tablespoon myrrh resin

1 tablespoon plantain leaf

½ cup + 1 tablespoon olive oil

½ ounce beeswax

20 drops tea tree essential oil

10 drops each lemon and
   rosemary essential oils

Put all the herbs into a glass baking dish and add enough olive oil to cover the herbs 1 or 2 inches deep. Bake in the oven at 170 degrees F for 4 hours and then strain. Pour the strained oil into a saucepan and add the beeswax. Gently heat until the beeswax is melted, stirring continuously. Turn off the heat and pour into container of your choice. Add the essential oils. Apply to the boil 3 times a day without a lot of rubbing and allow the salve to slowly be absorbed.

## Boil Poultice

1 teaspoon goldenseal root powder

Mix with just enough water to create a paste and spread it over the boil and surrounding area. Leave it on for 30 minutes. You can apply gentle heat over the poultice to attempt to bring the boil to a head.

# ≡ BRAIN FATIGUE ≡

Some days the brain just doesn't seem to fire at will like it used it. Instead of grabbing another cup of coffee, try one of these natural brain boosters.

## Brain-Boost Tea

1 ounce ashwagandha root

½ ounce holy basil leaf

1 ounce peppermint leaf

¼ ounce ginger root

Mix the herbs in a bowl and store in a glass jar. Steep 1 or 2 teaspoons in 10 ounces of hot water, covered, for 10 minutes. Drink 2 to 3 cups per day for 3 to 6 weeks, or as needed.

## Brain-Alive Tincture

1 teaspoon ginkgo leaf

1 teaspoon gotu kola leaf

1 teaspoon ashwagandha root

1½ teaspoons nettle leaf

½ teaspoon guarana nut

2 ounces vodka

Put the herbs in a 2-ounce glass jar. Cover with vodka, close tightly, and shake well. Keep in a cupboard or pantry for 3 weeks, shaking daily. Strain and transfer to a dropper bottle. Take 2 dropperfuls twice daily.

## Brain-Alert Essential Oil Blend

5 milliliters rosemary essential oil

2.5 milliliters ginger essential oil

2.5 milliliters lemon essential oil

Mix all the oils together in a 10-milliliter essential oil bottle with dropper cap. Drop 1 or 2 drops into your palms, rub them together, and take a few deep inhalations as needed.

# ≡ BRUISES ≡

A bruise is an injury to the blood vessels just below the skin causing a discoloration. Oils and liniments can promote healing. Because liniments typically work to break apart stagnation and because the collapse of blood vessels due to bruising results in stagnation of blood, an herbal liniment works well for bruising.

## Bruise Liniment

2 tablespoons comfrey leaf

2 tablespoons chamomile flower

1 tablespoon mullein flower

1 tablespoon calendula flower

$\frac{1}{16}$ teaspoon cayenne powder

2 cups witch hazel extract

Put the herbs in a pint jar and add witch hazel extract to fill. Close and shake well. Keep in a cupboard or pantry for 3 weeks, shaking every day. Strain and transfer the liquid into a clean bottle. To use, douse a cotton ball or pad with the liniment and apply to the bruise 3 times a day.

## Bruise-Healing Oil

fresh arnica flower

fresh parsley leaf

fresh comfrey leaf

olive oil

essential oils (optional)

Pack a mason jar full with equal parts of these three fresh herbs and pour olive oil over them to the top of the jar. Close and shake well. Remove the lid and cover with muslin cloth secured by a rubber band. Set the jar in full sun for 2 or 3 weeks. You will need a consistent temperature above 75 degrees F for best results, the warmer the better. Each day, remove the muslin cloth, put the lid on and shake the contents of the jar, and then replace the muslin. The muslin allows for water evaporation from the fresh plant material. Strain the herbs and transfer the oil into a clear bottle or jar. Add essential oils such as chamomile and cypress to give the oil a longer shelf life. Since you need fresh plant material and arnica flowers are available only once per year, you want your supply to last as long as possible. Rub the oil gently into the bruise and reapply as often as needed until the bruise heals.

# ⇒ CIRCULATION ⇐

Circulation comprises all of the pathways of the blood. It is directed by the pumping of the heart, which generates force to push the blood throughout the body. Sometimes smaller vessels become compromised, collapse, or are compressed by surrounding tissues. Other times if the heart isn't pumping with the same force it once was, it can be harder to get the blood to distal locations. This can lead to what is called poor circulation. The result is cold hands and feet, varicose veins, fatigue, and numbness and tingling.

## Healthy-Circulation Tonic Tea

*Taking a circulation tonic can support the system by toning the vessels and opening channels that may be compromised.*

1 ounce hawthorn berry

1 ounce bilberry fruit

½ ounce hawthorn leaf and flower

½ ounce ginkgo leaf

½ ounce horse chestnut

½ ounce ginger root

Mix the herbs in a bowl and store in a glass jar. Use 4 to 5 tablespoons to make 1-quart batches. Drink 1 to 3 cups per day for 8 to 12 weeks if desiring a tonic effect. Alternatively, you can drink 1 cup as desired for intermittent circulation support.

## Healthy-Circulation Tincture

1 teaspoon hawthorn berry

1 teaspoon bilberry fruit

½ teaspoon hawthorn leaf and flower

½ teaspoon ginkgo leaf

½ teaspoon horse chestnut

½ teaspoon ginger root

2 ounces vodka

Put the herbs in a 2-ounce glass jar. Cover with vodka, close, and shake well. Keep in a cupboard or pantry for 3 weeks, shaking every day. Strain and transfer to a dropper bottle. Take 2 dropperfuls twice daily.

# Cold-Hands/Feet Tincture

*I accidently discovered the powerful effects of lobelia on circulation one cold winter day. Our furnace had decided to go kaput and I could not get warm. I'd read about lobelia plenty, and because of its emetic warnings I'd always stayed away from it. But something was drawing me to it and as anyone who is guided by intuition will tell you, sometimes you just have to do something even when you can't logically explain it. So I opened the dropper bottle and put 10 drops of lobelia tincture under my tongue. Wow! Within minutes I could feel my body warming up, even all the way down to my toes!*

1 tablespoon ginkgo leaf

1 tablespoon hawthorn leaf and flower

1 teaspoon ginger root

½ teaspoon lobelia leaf

2 cups vodka

Put all the herbs in a pint jar and fill to the top with vodka. Close tightly and shake well. Keep in a cupboard or pantry for 2 to 3 weeks, shaking every day. Strain and transfer to a dropper bottle. Take 1 dropperful as needed.


# Cold-Feet Balm

2 tablespoons angelica root

1 tablespoon thyme leaf

1 tablespoon cinnamon chips

⅛ teaspoon cayenne powder

¾ cup olive oil

½ ounce beeswax

20 drops ginger essential oil

Put all the herbs in a glass baking dish and add enough olive oil to cover the herbs 1 or 2 inches deep. Bake at 170 degrees F for 4 hours. Allow to cool and then strain. Pour the oil into a saucepan and add the beeswax. Gently heat until the beeswax is melted. Pour into container of your choice and add the essential oil. Rub onto your feet, or better yet, get someone else to do it—by the fire, as you sip herbal tea.

# ≡ COLD SORES ≡

These painful blisters most often occur on the mouth and besides being itchy and sore, they can cause a lot of unnecessary self-deprecation. The stigma that goes along with cold sores can be unbearable, causing some to stay hidden away at home until an outbreak has healed. Caused by a virus that stays in the body, a cold sore can arise anytime the immune system is compromised—when you are stressed, sick, or overexerting yourself.

## Topical Lysine-Based Salve

1 tablespoon echinacea root

1 tablespoon lemon balm leaf

1 tablespoon St. John's wort leaf

1 tablespoon peppermint leaf

¾ cup olive oil

½ ounce beeswax

20 drops basil essential oil

40 drops melissa essential oil

Put all the herbs in a glass baking dish and add enough olive oil to cover the herbs 1 or 2 inches deep. Bake at 170 degrees F for 4 hours. Allow to cool and then strain. Pour the oil into a saucepan and add the beeswax. Gently heat until the beeswax is melted. Pour into container of your choice and add essential oils. Apply as needed.

## Outbreak-Quelling Tincture

1 teaspoon lomatium root

1 teaspoon lemon balm leaf

1 teaspoon St. John's wort leaf and flower

1 teaspoon spilanthes leaf and flower

2 ounces vodka

Put the herbs in a 2-ounce jar and add vodka to fill. Close tightly and shake well. Keep in a pantry or cupboard for 3 weeks, shaking every day. Strain and transfer to a dropper bottle. At the first tingle of a possible outbreak, begin taking 2 dropperfuls 4 times a day.

# ≡ CONCUSSION ≡

A concussion is a brain injury. It is caused by a blow to the head that actually causes the brain to rattle against the inside of the skull. As you can guess, this often leads to swelling and inflammation.

## Concussion-Treatment Fomentation

*Make a strong herbal brew to soak a towel in for topical application to the head. As it works to calm inflammation, it also feels good to the patient.*

1 ounce yucca root

1 ounce frankincense resin

1 ounce devil's club root

½ ounce ginger root

½ ounce turmeric root

8 cups water

Put all the herbs in a stockpot and add the water. Bring to a boil and reduce by a quarter. Strain out the herbs and then soak a towel in the warm brew. Wring out and apply to the head. Reapply often.

## Arnica Oil Concussion Treatment

*Arnica oil is a must for a concussion situation.*

freshly harvested arnica flowers

olive oil

Fill a quart mason jar with the flowers and fill to the top with olive oil. Close and shake well. Remove the lid and cover with muslin cloth secured by a rubber band. Set the jar in full sun for 2 to 3 weeks. You will need a consistent temperature above 75 degrees F for best results, the warmer the better. Each day, remove the muslin cloth and close with the lid, shake the contents of the jar, and then replace the muslin. The muslin allows for water evaporation from the fresh plant material. Strain the herbs and transfer the oil into a clear bottle or jar. Generously apply to the area of injury and all surrounding areas.

# ARNICA TINCTURE FOR SERIOUS BODILY INJURY

Arnica tincture is toxic and is therefore not recommended in this book, nor is it readily available over the counter. But it can be extremely beneficial in times of serious bodily injury. Please consult with your naturopath or certified herbal practitioner on how to use 2 to 3 **drops** to treat concussion or other significant trauma such as a car accident or childbirth.

## Concussion-Treatment Tincture

½ teaspoon turmeric root

½ teaspoon white willow bark

½ teaspoon cat's claw bark

½ teaspoon lavender flower

¹⁄₁₆ teaspoon cayenne powder

2 ounces vodka

Put the herbs in a 2-ounce jar and add vodka to fill. Close tightly and shake well. Keep in a pantry or cupboard for 3 weeks, shaking every day. Strain and transfer to a dropper bottle. Take 2 dropperfuls 3 times a day for 2 weeks.

## ═ CONSTIPATION ═

We all have days when things don't flow as normal. Consider these recipes for acute and chronic types of constipation.

## Unclogging Tea

2 ounces fenugreek seed

1 ounce alder buckthorn bark

½ ounce slippery elm bark

½ ounce marshmallow bark

Mix the herbs in a bowl and store in a jar. When needed, make tea by the cup. Simmer 1 or 2 teaspoons in 12 ounces of hot water, covered, for 10 minutes. Strain and drink hot. I prefer to drink this tea before bed so it gently works while I sleep.

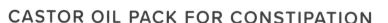

# CASTOR OIL PACK FOR CONSTIPATION

This is a simple topical treatment that has profound effects on the body. Spread 2 to 3 tablespoons of castor oil on the abdomen, ensuring to cover the entire area. Next place an old cotton t-shirt or towel over the abdomen. Be sure it is something you are not that attached to, as the castor oil will stain it. Then place a hot water bottle or heating pad over the towel and relax for 30 minutes. This treatment works best if done a minimum of 4 consecutive days a week.

## Chronic-Constipation Capsules

*This is a reprint of Dr. John Christopher's recipe for lower bowel tonic. When tone has diminished, the natural propulsion of waste stops. If chronic constipation has been present for a long time, it may take up to 20 capsules per day to break through the blockages and tone the lower intestine.*

1 ounce cascara sagrada bark powder

⅛ ounce barberry bark powder

⅛ ounce cayenne powder

⅛ ounce ginger root powder

⅛ ounce goldenseal root powder

⅛ ounce lobelia leaf or seed powder

⅛ ounce raspberry leaf powder

⅛ ounce turkey rhubarb root powder

⅛ ounce fennel powder

Mix the powders in a bowl and fill 200 empty capsules. Begin taking 7 or 8 capsules 3 times a day for 1 or 2 weeks and then reduce the daily amount slowly.

## ═ DIARRHEA ═

Diarrhea can come on from many causes. It can be acute from a bacterial or viral infection or from spoiled food or water. It can also take a chronic form caused by stress, a low-grade infection, or improper digestive flora. One thing to always keep in mind when diarrhea strikes is the need to stay hydrated. Diarrhea is extremely dehydrating, as it pulls enormous amounts of water from the body.

# Acute-Diarrhea Tincture

1 teaspoon Oregon grape root

1 teaspoon goldenseal root

1 teaspoon licorice root

2 teaspoons raspberry leaf

2 ounces vodka or apple cider vinegar

Put the herbs in a 2-ounce jar and add vodka or apple cider vinegar to fill. Close tightly and shake well. Keep in a pantry or cupboard for 3 weeks, shaking every day. Strain and transfer to a 2-ounce dropper bottle. Take 2 dropperfuls 3 times a day for 3 to 5 days when diarrhea strikes. Continue taking 1 day past the resolution of symptoms.

# Hiker's Anti-Diarrhea Tincture

*I've received many phone calls over the years from friends who have returned from amazing backpacking trips only to have a bout of diarrhea. This formula is targeted to stop the diarrhea and also kill any bacteria that may be causing it.*

1 teaspoon wormwood leaf

1 teaspoon usnea, chopped up

1 teaspoon pau d'arco bark

1 teaspoon yarrow flower

1 teaspoon slippery elm bark

½ teaspoon Oregon grape root

½ teaspoon cinnamon bark

4 ounces vodka or apple cider vinegar

Put the herbs in a 4-ounce jar and add vodka or apple cider vinegar to fill. Close tightly and shake well. Keep in a pantry or cupboard for 3 weeks, shaking every day. Strain and transfer to a dropper bottle. Take 2 dropperfuls 3 times a day for 3 to 5 days when diarrhea strikes. Continue taking 3 days past the resolution of symptoms.

# Intestine-Calming Essential Oil Blend

*This blend has proven to calm the overactivity of the lower intestines.*

20 drops frankincense essential oil

20 drops chamomile essential oil

10 drops fennel essential oil

5 drops lavender essential oil

4 ounces hemp oil

Blend all ingredients in a 4-ounce bottle. Rub 1 to 2 teaspoons into the skin of the abdomen when needed.

# ≡ DIZZINESS ≡

Sometimes dizziness is virally induced after a cold, sometimes it is structurally related or stems from hypoglycemia, and sometimes it comes on for no good reason. Whatever the cause, dizziness can be troublesome. The following herbal suggestions have proven helpful, but if you try these and they don't work, consider finding someone who treats vertigo with the Epley maneuver.

## Rose Anti-Dizziness Tea

*Drinking rose petal tea for dizziness is an old nature cure.*

1 teaspoon dried rose petals
8 ounces of water

Heat the water to boiling and steep the petals for 8 minutes, covered. Drink 3 cups a day as needed.

## Anti-Dizziness Tincture

1 teaspoon nettle leaf
1 teaspoon alfalfa leaf
1 teaspoon hawthorn leaf

1 teaspoon echinacea root
2 ounces vodka

Put the herbs in a 2-ounce jar and add vodka to fill. Close tightly and shake well. Keep in a pantry or cupboard for 3 weeks, shaking every day. Strain and transfer to a 2-ounce dropper bottle. Take 1 dropperful as needed.

## Viral-Dizziness Tincture

1 teaspoon lemon balm leaf
1 teaspoon lomatium root
1 teaspoon St. John's wort leaf and flower

1 teaspoon ashwagandha root
2 ounces vodka

Put the herbs in a 2-ounce jar and add vodka to fill. Close tightly and shake well. Keep in a pantry or cupboard for 3 weeks, shaking every day. Strain and transfer to a 2-ounce dropper bottle. Take 1 to 2 dropperfuls every 4 hours until symptoms subside.

See also "Earaches" in the "Immune Defense" section. Many things—including colds, wax buildup, and pressure caused by airplane flights or elevation gain—can affect our ears. As a practitioner I often see eardrums that have been ruptured by treating the ears overaggressively. Remember that there is a membrane in the ear canal (the eardrum) that is a protective barrier between the external ear and the eustachian tube, and do your best not to poke at it or drive wax in too deep using such things as Q-tips and fingers.

## Wax-Breakdown Oil

¼ cup olive oil
1 clove garlic

Warm the garlic clove in the olive oil on low for 1 hour, covered. Strain out the clove and drip 1 or 2 drops of the oil into the ear and massage. Do this daily for 7 days, and the wax should loosen up enough to come out on its own. You can also try flushing out the wax after 7 days by filling an irrigation syringe with slightly warm water and forcefully squirting it into the ear.

# TINNITUS TREATMENT

Tinnitus is a perception of ringing or roaring in the ears when no sound is present externally. For relief, wrap a tiny pinch of asafoetida in a tiny bit of paper towel and insert into your ear while sleeping. Be careful to not insert too deeply.

# ≡ ECZEMA ≡

Eczema is a condition that often results in scaly, itchy, peeling skin. Sometimes it can create small blisters filled with fluid. In my experience, eczema seems to be caused by an external allergic reaction, stress, or food allergies resulting in digestive imbalance. I worked with a dear friend for years to try to identify the cause of her eczema. We went all the normal routes with herbs and supplements, and finally we identified it as an allergic reaction to beeswax. I encourage you to find a practitioner who will run the gamut with you to identify the source; the relief is well worth the investigation. In the meantime, here are a couple of recipes to calm the inflammation.

## Eczema-Calming Wash

1 ounce plantain leaf

1 ounce comfrey leaf

1 ounce slippery elm bark

1 ounce calendula flowers

Mix the herbs in a bowl and store in a glass jar. When needed, put 5 tablespoons in a quart jar and pour boiling water over the herbs to fill the jar. Let steep 1 hour and then strain. You can keep the herbs to reuse. Either pour the brew into a bowl and soak the affected area or soak a cotton cloth and wrap the area. Treat for 20 to 30 minutes once or twice daily for temporary relief.

## Eczema-Calming Salve

1 tablespoon plantain leaf

1 tablespoon comfrey leaf

1 tablespoon elderflower

1 tablespoon chickweed leaf

¾ cup olive oil

30 drops chamomile essential oil

5–10 drops balsam essential oil

Put the herbs in a glass baking dish and add enough oil to cover the herbs 1 or 2 inches deep. Bake in the oven at 170 degrees F for 4 hours. Allow to cool slightly and then strain the herbs from the oil. Pour the oil into a saucepan and add the beeswax. Gently warm the oil until the wax is completely melted. Be sure to stir continuously. Pour into container of your choice and add the essential oils. Apply as needed.

Our handy modern technology is truly taking a toll on our eyes. Combine this with being over the age of forty and it's a double assault. I honestly thought it was crazy when all my friends began needing reading glasses. For almost a year, I lived in complete denial that my eyes were having difficulty reading smaller text, including on my phone. I'd seen the larger print books at the library and thought that was only for people over eighty. Ha! Well, I still refuse to wear reading glasses or turn on a larger font for my text messages, but I also now religiously take my eye tonics.

## Eye-Strengthening Syrup

1 ounce bilberry fruit

1 ounce ginkgo leaf

1 ounce triphala

½ ounce rosehips

½ ounce fennel seed

8 cups water

3 cups cane sugar or honey

¼ cup apple cider vinegar

Put the herbs in a saucepan with the water. Bring to a boil and reduce by half on a medium-low heat. Strain the out herbs and put the brew back in the pan. Add sugar or honey and gently heat to mix if necessary, stirring continuously. Turn off the heat, add apple cider vinegar, and allow to cool. Transfer to container of your choice and store in the refrigerator. Take 1 teaspoon once or twice daily.

## Screen Time Relief Mask

1 ounce bentonite clay

1 teaspoon chickweed leaf powder

1 teaspoon lavender flower powder

Mix all ingredients together and store in a glass jar. When feeling the effects of too much screen time, mix 2 teaspoons with just enough water to make a paste. Gently apply to eyelids and around eyebrows. Place two raw cucumber slices over your eyes and lie down for 20 minutes. Wash off with cool water.

## Excessive-Tearing Spray

40 milliliters rose water

10 milliliters previously prepared coleus tincture

10 milliliters previously prepared coriander seed tincture

Pour the rose water into a 2-ounce spray bottle and add the tinctures. Shake gently before spritzing. Spray into eyes and onto eyelids as needed and use a cotton ball to gently wipe away.

## QI GONG FOR YOUR EYES

Another great eye health tool is qi gong for the eyes. Find a comfortable place to sit and focus your eyes on something 2 to 3 feet in front of you. Then look up and focus on something 50 to 100 feet away. Hold the gaze on each thing for 1 minute, moving back and forth for 5 or 10 minutes. This strengthens the muscles and focusing factors of the eyes.

# ≡ FATIGUE ≡

Use the following general recipes to put a little extra bounce in your step. If fatigue presents as a sudden change or is chronic, it is best to consult your health care practitioner, just as for any sudden or chronic condition.

## Energy-Tonic Syrup

1 ounce licorice root

1 ounce eleuthero root

½ ounce alfalfa leaf

½ ounce nettle leaf

½ ounce yerba mate or guarana seed

3 cups raw cane sugar or honey

¼ cup apple cider vinegar

8 cups water

Put the herbs in a saucepan with the water. Bring to a boil and reduce by half on a medium-low heat. Strain the out herbs and put the brew back in the pan. Add sugar or honey and gently heat to mix if necessary, stirring continuously. Turn off the heat, add the apple cider vinegar, and allow to cool. Transfer to container of your choice and store in the refrigerator. Take 1 teaspoon as needed.

## Get-Up-and-Go Tea

1 ounce peppermint leaf

1 ounce spearmint leaf

½ ounce rosemary leaf

½ ounce ginkgo leaf

½ ounce lemongrass

½ ounce damiana leaf

Mix the herbs in a bowl and store in a glass jar. Make tea by the cup. Steep 1 or 2 teaspoons in 10 ounces of hot water, covered, for 10 minutes. Drink a cup as desired for an energy boost.

## Wake-Up Spritzer

*There is nothing more refreshing then a spritz to the face. It wakes us up and revives the soul.*

30 drops wild orange essential oil

20 drops basil essential oil

10 drops rosemary essential oil

2 ounces distilled water

Put the essential oils into a 2-ounce spray bottle and add distilled water to fill. Close and shake to mix well. Spray on the face or around the head as needed.

With more than three million cases reported a year, I think we can safely say gallstones are quite common these days. They are tiny stones formed in the gallbladder from hardened deposits of cholesterol, bile, or bilirubin. At times they also get stuck, which can lead to more serious conditions that should be treated right away.

## Gallbladder-Tonic Tea

*The bitter principle is what drives this formula and stimulates the dissolution process.*

1 ounce celandine leaf and flower

1 ounce olive leaf

1 ounce peppermint leaf

½ ounce dandelion root

½ ounce fennel seed

Mix the herbs in a bowl and store in a glass jar. Use 4 to 5 tablespoons to make 1-quart batches. Drink 3 cups per day for 6 to 8 weeks for a tonic effect.

## Gallbladder Tincture

1 teaspoon celandine leaf and flower

1 teaspoon olive leaf

1 teaspoon turmeric root

½ teaspoon dandelion root

½ teaspoon fennel seed

2 ounces vodka or apple cider

Put all the herbs in a 2-ounce jar and add vodka or apple cider vinegar to fill. Close tightly and shake well. Keep in a pantry or cupboard for 3 weeks, shaking every day. Strain and transfer to a 2-ounce dropper bottle. Take 1 dropperful 3 times a day for 8 to 12 weeks.

## Gallbladder Topical Treatment

1 ounce olive leaf

1 ounce lavender flower

8 ounces castor oil

40 drops lemon essential oil

25 drops rosemary essential oil

10 drops peppermint essential oil

Put the herbs and the castor oil into a glass baking dish and bake at 170 degrees F for 4 hours. Allow to slightly cool and then strain. Transfer to container of your choice and add the essential oils. Rub 2 tablespoons over the gallbladder area on the abdomen and surrounding areas. Cover with a cotton towel and then a hot water bottle or heating pad. Relax for 30 to 45 minutes, or put on before bed and go to sleep.

# ≡ GAS ≡

It can strike anytime. If gas is something you experience regularly, I'm here to say that isn't necessarily normal. While occasional gas is inevitable due to certain food choices, stress, or illness, gas shouldn't be a part of your regular daily experience. Typically this is a sign that you should examine. What makes it better or worse? When does it happen? Do your digestive system a favor and spend a bit of time examining the flatulence cycle.

## Gas-Relief Tea

1 ounce lemongrass

1½ ounces fennel seed

1¼ ounces marshmallow root

¼ ounce lavender flower

Mix the herbs in a bowl and store in a glass jar. Make tea by the cup. Steep 1 to 2 teaspoons in 10 ounces of hot water, covered, for 10 minutes. Drink as needed.

## Gas-Blaster Capsules

½ ounce slippery elm bark powder

¼ ounce fennel seed powder

¼ ounce coriander seed powder

¼ ounce catnip leaf powder

¼ ounce gentian root powder

Mix the powders in a bowl and fill 200 empty capsules. Take 2 capsules before each meal to reduce gas-creating opportunity.

# ≡ GUM DISEASE ≡

Whether due to lack of flossing, age, or simply genetics, some gum lines begin to recede faster than others. This can leave the mouth and teeth susceptible to a host of problems, including infections.

## Receding-Gum Rinse

*Use to tone gum tissue and encourage gum health.*

1 teaspoon sumac berry

1 teaspoon white oak bark

1 teaspoon myrrh resin

2 ounces vodka

Put the herbs in a 2-ounce jar and fill to the top with vodka. Close the jar tightly and shake well. Keep in a cupboard or pantry for 14 days, shaking daily. Strain and transfer to a 2-ounce dropper bottle. Add 1 or 2 dropperfuls to 1 ounce of water and swish in the mouth for 1 minute twice daily. Spit out afterward.

## Gingivitis Tincture

*Rinsing with this antibacterial tincture can give the gums just what they need to fight infection.*

1 teaspoon goldenseal root

1 teaspoon myrrh resin

1 teaspoon sumac berry

1 teaspoon calendula flower

2 ounces vodka

Put all the herbs in a 2-ounce jar and fill to the top with vodka. Close the jar tightly and shake well. Keep in a cupboard or pantry for 3 weeks, shaking every day. Strain and transfer to a 2-ounce dropper bottle. Swish twice daily with 3 dropperfuls mixed with 1 ounce of water.

See also "Allergies." My poor husband has suffered allergies his entire life. While I look forward to spring, summer, and early fall, my husband has a level of hesitation about welcoming the changes of the seasons due to his suffering. I celebrate the smell of freshly cut grass, but he wears a bandana to mow the lawn. I am constantly pushing remedies on him, and when he takes them he has a break from the allergic cough, runny nose, red eyes, and sneezing.

## Hay-Fever Eyewash

1 ounce nettle leaf

1 ounce calendula flower

1 ounce chickweed leaf

1 ounce eyebright leaf

Mix the herbs in a bowl and store in a glass jar. When needed, put 5 tablespoons in a pint jar and pour boiling water over the herbs to fill the jar. Let steep 1 hour and then strain. You can keep the herbs to reuse. Soak a cotton cloth in the infusion and douse the eye, inside and out, with it. Repeat 4 to 6 times a day.

## Hay-Fever Tea

1 ounce chamomile flower (purchased from a reputable source so that cross-contamination with ragweed is not an issue)

1 ounce peppermint leaf

½ ounce elderflower

½ ounce nettle leaf

Mix the herbs in a bowl and store in a glass jar. Make tea by the cup. Steep 1 or 2 teaspoons in 10 ounces of hot water, covered, for 10 minutes. Drink as needed or 3 cups a day during days of heightened pollen count.

## NETI POT FORMULA FOR HAY FEVER

Add 10 drops spikenard tincture to the usual water and salt, as it is a powerful aid to the upper respiratory system.

# ≡ HEADACHE ≡

These recipes help with simple tension headaches.

## Rose-Vinegar Headache Compress

**fresh rose petals**
**white or apple cider vinegar**

Stuff a 1-pint jar almost full of fresh rose petals and fill to the top with vinegar. Close the lid and shake gently. Keep in a cupboard or pantry for 14 days, gently shaking daily. Strain and transfer to container of your choice. When needed, soak a cotton cloth in the solution and apply to either the forehead or the nape of the neck.

## Headache-Relief Oil

**1 ounce fresh poplar buds**
**1 ounce lavender flower**

**¾ cup olive oil**

Put both herbs in a glass baking dish and add enough olive oil to cover the herbs 1 or 2 inches deep. Bake at 170 degrees F for 4 hours. Allow to cool and then strain. Pour the oil into container of your choice. When needed, rub 1 teaspoon onto the temples or the nape of the neck.

## Headache-Relief Tincture

**2 teaspoons fennel seed**
**1 teaspoon white willow bark**
**1 teaspoon California poppy
  leaf and flower**

**1 teaspoon licorice root**
**2 ounces vodka or apple cider vinegar**

Put the herbs in a 2-ounce jar and add vodka or apple cider vinegar to fill. Close tightly and shake well. Keep in a pantry or cupboard for 3 weeks, shaking every day. Strain and transfer to a 2-ounce dropper bottle. Take 1 to 2 dropperfuls every 20 minutes until pain subsides. If you need to exceed 6 doses, consider another treatment.

# ≡ HEAT EXHAUSTION ≡

Hydration and electrolyte replenishing are important steps to treat heat exhaustion. Also helpful is using essential oils to encourage the body to relax and mobilize the parasympathetic system to regain balance.

## Hydration Tea

2 ounces lemon balm leaf

1 ounce rosehips

½ ounce nettle leaf

½ ounce chickweed leaf

1 teaspoon salt

Mix the herbs and the salt in a bowl and store in a glass jar. Make tea by the cup (using 2 teaspoons, steeping for 10 minutes) or the quart (using 4 tablespoons, steeping 1 or 2 hours). Drink as needed, hot or cold.

## Essential Oil Blend for Heat Exhaustion

6 milliliters basil essential oil

2 milliliters eucalyptus essential oil

2 milliliters geranium essential oil

Blend the oils in a 10-milliliter essential oil bottle. Drop 1 or 2 drops on the palms and take a few deep inhalations as needed, or add to an essential oil diffuser.

# ≡ HEMORRHOIDS ≡

Hemorrhoids occur in varying degrees but all should be treated. Understanding the difference between hemorrhoids and fissures is important so that you are treating correctly. A hemorrhoid occurs when one of the vascular cushions in the anal canal becomes irritated, inflamed, and/or swollen, and as it worsens it can swell outside of the anus. A fissure is a laceration or cut anywhere along the anus. The latter tends to itch and can bleed bright red drops into the toilet bowl, whereas hemorrhoids tend to be painful and blood is more often seen upon wiping.

## Hemorrhoid Comfort Salve

2 ounces comfrey leaf

1 ounce plantain leaf

1 ounce yarrow flower

¾ cup olive oil

½ ounce beeswax

20–40 drops lavender essential oil

Put the herbs in a glass baking dish and add enough oil to cover the herbs 1 or 2 inches deep. Bake at 170 degrees F for 4 hours. Allow to cool and then strain. Pour the oil into a saucepan and add the beeswax. Gently heat until the beeswax is melted. Pour into container of your choice and add essential oil as desired. Apply as needed.

## Fomentation for Topical Hemorrhoid Treatment

1½ ounces yarrow flower

1 ounce chamomile flower

1 ounce calendula flower

1 ounce burdock root

Mix the herbs in a bowl and store in a glass jar. When needed, put 6 tablespoons in a quart jar and pour boiling water over the herbs to fill the jar. Let steep 1 or 2 hours, or overnight, and then strain. You can keep the herbs to reuse. Gently warm the infusion and soak a cotton cloth in it. Wring out well and apply for 20 to 30 minutes once or twice daily for temporary relief.

## Hemorrhoid Healing Pads

1¼ cups witch hazel extract

½ cup aloe vera gel

15 drops lavender essential oil

cotton pads

Mix the witch hazel extract, aloe vera gel, and lavender oil in a bowl and put into a large ziplock freezer bag. Add the cotton pads and shake around until they are saturated. Keep in the refrigerator and apply 1 to 3 daily to the affected area. Many of my patients prefer to simply tuck them in and leave them to rest.

# ⟹ HIVES ⟹

Hives can appear as raised, red, and perhaps circular bumps on the skin. Rarely is there just one. Sometimes they itch, burn, or sting. They are usually triggered by an allergic reaction, although stress or a virus are also common causes.

## Tincture for Allergic Hives

1 tablespoon nettle leaf

1 tablespoon rosehips

½ teaspoon St. John's wort leaf and flower

½ teaspoon echinacea root

2 ounces vodka or apple cider vinegar

Put the herbs in a 2-ounce jar and add vodka or apple cider vinegar to fill. Close tightly and shake well. Keep in a pantry or cupboard for 3 weeks, shaking every day. Strain and transfer to a 2-ounce dropper bottle. Take 1 to 2 dropperfuls 3 times a day when needed.

## Topical Wash for Hives

1 ounce chamomile flower

1 ounce plantain lea

1 ounce comfrey leaf

1 ounce elderflower

Mix the herbs in a bowl and store in a glass jar. When needed, put 6 tablespoon in a quart jar and pour boiling water over the herbs to fill the jar. Let steep 1 or 2 hours, or overnight, and then strain. You can keep the herbs to reuse. Use the solution at a cool temperature. Soak a cotton cloth, wring it out, and wrap the area. You can also douse the area with a drenched cotton ball or submerge the area in the infusion. Treat for 20 or 30 minutes once or twice daily for temporary relief.

## Hives-Relief Spray

*Make a batch of this ahead of time and keep it on hand for sudden flare-ups.*

1 tablespoon plantain leaf

1 tablespoon white oak bark

1 teaspoon calendula flower

2 ounces apple cider vinegar

Put the herbs in a 2-ounce jar and add apple cider vinegar to fill. Close tightly and shake well. Keep in a pantry or cupboard for 3 weeks, shaking every day. Strain and transfer to a 2-ounce spray bottle. Spritz as needed.

## ═ HOARSENESS ═

A change in voice is typically a clear sign that your body is defending itself, unless you've been singing regularly, in which case it's a sign of fatigue. These remedies can help either way.

### Back-to-Voice Tea

1 ounce thyme leaf

1 ounce marshmallow root

1 ounce elderberry

½ ounce wild cherry bark

½ ounce yerba santa leaf

Mix the herbs in a bowl and store in a glass jar. Make tea by the cup. Steep 1 or 2 teaspoons in 10 ounces of hot water, covered, for 10 minutes. Drink as needed.

### Throat Rub for Hoarseness

2 tablespoons cleavers leaf and flower

1 tablespoon rose petals

½ cup olive oil

10–15 drops frankincense essential oil

Put the herbs in a glass baking dish and add enough olive oil to cover the herbs 1 or 2 inches deep. Bake at 170 degrees F for 4 hours. Allow to cool and then strain. Add the essential oil and transfer to container of your choice. Rub a bit externally onto the throat as needed.

## MARSHMALLOW OR LICORICE ROOT FOR HOARSENESS

Take small pieces of marshmallow root or licorice root to suck on. Their natural moisture-producing and soothing properties go a long way.

Our body needs energy, and we get that energy from the food we eat. When we haven't eaten enough or it's been too long since our last meal, our blood sugar dips low. This can cause dizziness, headache, nausea, fatigue, and/or an overall sense of blah. Have this tea on hand to ensure blood sugar stays balanced throughout the day, and keep the tincture around for acute situations.

## Blood-Sugar-Balancing Tea

1 ounce alfalfa leaf

1 ounce hibiscus flower

¾ ounce nettle leaf

½ ounce comfrey leaf

½ ounce horsetail

¼ ounce ginger root

Mix the herbs in a bowl and store in a glass jar. Make tea by the cup. Steep 1 or 2 teaspoons in 10 ounces of hot water, covered, for 10 minutes. Drink as needed or twice daily between meals.

## Blood-Sugar-Balancing Tincture

2 teaspoons licorice root

1 teaspoon nettle leaf

1 teaspoon raspberry leaf

1 teaspoon fennel seed

2 ounces apple cider vinegar

Put the herbs in a 2-ounce jar and add apple cider vinegar to fill. Close tightly and shake well. Keep in a pantry or cupboard for 3 weeks, shaking every day. Strain and transfer to a 2-ounce dropper bottle. Take 1 dropperful between meals.

# ≡ INCONTINENCE ≡

Incontinence is the inability to hold one's bladder, and it is a growing epidemic. As our food becomes less mineral dense, the tone and strength of our ligament systems are greatly affected. Kegels and other pelvic floor exercises are helpful, but essential nutrients are necessary, as is identifying bladder irritants that worsen the condition. In my experience, caffeine and certain foods are culprits.

## Bladder-Tonic Tincture

1 teaspoon goldenrod leaf and flower

1 teaspoon pipsissewa leaf and flower

½ teaspoon raspberry leaf

½ teaspoon burdock root

½ teaspoon chickweed leaf and flower

2 ounces vodka

Put the herbs in a 2-ounce jar and add vodka to fill. Close tightly and shake well. Keep in a pantry or cupboard for 3 weeks, shaking every day. Strain and transfer to a 2-ounce dropper bottle. Take 1 dropperful 3 times a day for 8 to 12 weeks.

## Bladder-Tone Topical Strengthener

20 drops copiaba essential oil

5 drops cypress essential oil

2 ounces castor oil

Mix the ingredients and rub a small amount into the area on the abdomen above the bladder once daily.

Indigestion can be gas, bloating, heartburn, acid reflux, water brash, or excessive burping. As a culture we've decided many of these symptoms are normal, but they don't have to be. With minor dietary shifts and changes to eating habits, all of these can diminish and go away.

## Digest-Aid Capsules

½ ounce fennel seed powder

½ ounce caraway seed powder

½ ounce marshmallow root powder

½ ounce catnip powder

Mix the powdered herbs in a bowl and fill 200 empty capsules. Take 2 capsules with each meal. Also see the recipe for Appetite-Stimulating Bitters under "Appetite, Decreased"—a great aperitif for anyone who experiences regular indigestion after eating.

## Heartburn-Easing Capsules

½ ounce fennel seed powder

½ ounce ginger root powder

½ ounce slippery elm bark power

½ ounce skullcap leaf powder

Mix the powdered herbs in a bowl and fill 200 empty capsules. Take 2 capsules with each meal.

## Indigestion Castor-Oil Rub

2 tablespoons chamomile flower

1 tablespoon coriander seed

1 tablespoon lemon balm leaf

1 cup castor oil

40 drops lavendar essential oil (optional)

Put the herbs in a glass baking dish and add enough castor oil to cover the herbs 1 or 2 inches deep. Bake at 170 degrees F for 4 hours. Allow to cool and then strain. Transfer to container of your choice and add the essential oil if desired. Rub 2 tablespoons over the stomach area. Cover with a cotton towel and then a hot water bottle or heating pad. Relax for 30 to 45 minutes, or put on before bed and go to sleep.

# HACKS FOR EXCESS STOMACH ACID

If excess stomach acid is an issue for you, please consider the following:

- If you use acid blockers, you are eliminating the first step in the natural digestive process, which can lead to chronic digestive inflammation. Try to identify the cause of excess stomach acid so you can wean yourself from them.

- Consider an anti-inflammatory diet for 3 weeks. You may be surprised how easy it is to identify what causes your acid reflux, heartburn, or stomach upset.

- Ensure you are hydrated.

- Try using digestive enzymes with each meal for a while to retrain your digestive system.

- Eat slowly.

- Look at and smell your food before you eat it. This may sound silly, but both of these actions give your body signals to turn on the digestive process.

# ≡ INSOMNIA ≡

Whether chronic or arising out of nowhere, insomnia will make the following day challenging. Investigating and understanding the cause of your insomnia is key to treating it. If stress has spiked and insomnia has arrived with it, nervines are necessary to calm the overstimulated state. If stress and insomnia have plagued you for years, consider herbal adrenal support. If hormonal changes have accompanied insomnia, using herbs to balance the liver and hormonal system is the best place to start. See the following recipes and start with the simplest first, as gentle shifts often have profound effects.

## Bedtime Tea

1 ounce anise seed

2 ½ ounces passionflower leaf and flower

¼ ounce hop strobiles

¼ ounce ginger root

Mix the herbs in a bowl and store in a glass jar. Make tea by the cup. Steep 1 or 2 teaspoons in 10 ounces of hot water, covered, for 10 minutes. Drink 1 hour before bed.

## Acute Insomnia Relaxation Tincture

1 teaspoon hop strobiles

1 teaspoon valerian root

1 teaspoon California poppy
  leaf and flower

2 teaspoons ashwagandha root

2 ounces vodka or apple cider vinegar

Put the herbs in a 2-ounce jar and add vodka or apple cider vinegar to fill. Close tightly and shake well. Keep in a pantry or cupboard for 3 weeks, shaking every day. Strain and transfer to a 2-ounce dropper bottle. Take 2 dropperfuls 30 minutes before bed and then 1 more when you lie down to sleep.

# Hormonally Influenced Insomnia Tincture

1½ teaspoons skullcap leaf

1 teaspoon rhodiola root bark

½ teaspoon ashwagandha root

½ teaspoon partridge berry

½ teaspoon angelica root

2 ounces vodka or apple cider vinegar

Put the herbs in a 2-ounce jar and add vodka or apple cider vinegar to fill. Close tightly and shake well. Keep in a pantry or cupboard for 3 weeks, shaking every day. Strain and transfer to a 2-ounce dropper bottle. Take 1 dropperful 3 times a day for 8 to 12 weeks.

# Nervine Insomnia Tonic Tincture

1 teaspoon chamomile leaf

1 teaspoon skullcap leaf

1 teaspoon black cohosh root

½ teaspoon wood betony leaf

½ teaspoon nettle leaf

2 ounces vodka or apple cider vinegar

Put the herbs in a 2-ounce jar and add vodka or apple cider vinegar to fill. Close tightly and shake well. Keep in a pantry or cupboard for 3 weeks, shaking every day. Strain and transfer to a 2-ounce dropper bottle. Take 1 dropperful 3 times a day for 8 to 12 weeks.

# Nighttime Sleep Salve

1 tablespoon hop strobiles

1 tablespoon lemon balm leaf

1 tablespoon St. John's wort
  leaf and flower

1 tablespoon rose petals

¾ cup olive oil

½ ounce beeswax

20–40 drops lavender essential oil

Put the herbs in a glass baking dish and cover with olive oil to a depth of 1 or 2 inches. Bake at 170 degrees F for 4 hours. Allow to cool and then strain. Pour oil into a saucepan and add the beeswax. Gently heat until the beeswax is melted. Pour into container of your choice and add lavender essential oil. Rub into your temples and the nape of your neck each night before bed.

# ⇒ KIDNEY STONES ⇐

The kidneys are among the most important organs of the human body, and their job is to filter liquid waste. It is a small-channeled and delicate system not made for solid particles such as stones. This is why it can be excruciating when kidney stones arise, as the pathways are too small for passage.

## Stone-Relief Tincture

1 teaspoon turmeric root

½ teaspoon stone breaker leaf

½ teaspoon pipsissewa leaf

½ teaspoon hydrangea root

½ teaspoon ginger root

½ teaspoon parsley root

2 ounces vodka

Put the herbs in a 2-ounce jar and add vodka to fill. Close tightly and shake well. Keep in a pantry or cupboard for 3 weeks, shaking every day. Strain and transfer to a 2-ounce dropper bottle. As a preventive measure but for short-term use, take 1 dropperful 1 or 2 times a day. For acute symptoms, take 2 dropperfuls every 3 to 4 hours.

## Stone-Relief Capsules

¾ ounce turmeric root powder

¼ ounce stone breaker leaf powder

¼ ounce pipsissewa leaf powder

¼ ounce hydrangea root powder

¼ ounce ginger root powder

¼ ounce parsley root powder

Mix the powdered herbs in a bowl and fill 200 empty capsules. Take 2 twice per day or for acute pain, 2 every 3 hours.

# ≡ KITCHEN BURNS ≡

They are inevitable. As I teach my children to cook and bake, I already dread the day they'll get their first kitchen burn. It always feels so personal and just hurts so bad. Luckily these handy herbs make a big difference.

## Lavender Burn Balm

*Such an easy one to have handy.*

**1–2 drops lavender essential oil**

Apply oil right on the burn to relieve the heat and sting.

## Kitchen-Burn Salve

**1 tablespoon comfrey leaf**
**1 tablespoon chickweed leaf**
**1 tablespoon plantain leaf**
**1 tablespoon St. John's wort**
**leaf and flower**

**¾ cup olive oil**
**½ ounce beeswax**
**40 drops lavender or lemon**
**balm essential oil**

Put the herbs in a glass baking dish and cover with olive oil to a depth of 1 or 2 inches. Bake at 170 degrees F for 4 hours. Allow to cool and then strain. Pour the oil into a saucepan and add the beeswax. Gently heat until the beeswax is melted. Pour into container of your choice and add the essential oil. Apply as needed to relieve the sting and help the burn heal.

# NATUROPATHIC WOUND HEALING

Decrease your chance of scar tissue from a wound by keeping it completely covered with salve consistently. When you keep the area moist with healing agents, it will heal from the inside out. Allowing a scab to form from drying out actually expedites tissue death, allowing scar tissue to form.

## Herbal Ice Cubes for Burns

**2 tablespoons lavender flower**  **2 tablespoons chamomile flower**

Add the herbs to a pint jar and fill with hot water. Let this steep overnight. In the morning, strain out the herbs, pour the infusion into an ice cube tray, and freeze. Appy cubes to burns as needed.

## ⟩⟩⟩ LUMBAGO ⟨⟨⟨

Lower back pain limits our daily activities and is best not ignored. Consult an acupuncturist, naturopath, massage therapist, or chiropractor to investigate the source of the problem if unknown. If due to an acute injury, baby yourself until well after your symptoms are relieved.

## Topical Warming Pack

**1 tablespoon white mustard powder**  **castor oil**
**½ cup oatstraw powder**

Mix the ingredients in a bowl with enough room temperature water to make a paste. Do not use hot water as it will release the oils in the mustard that we want to preserve. Put the paste on a large piece of plastic wrap and fold it over to completely cover the paste and make a nice square or rectangle the size of the area you will be treating. Set it aside on top of a hot water bottle or heating pad. Rub a bit of castor oil into the treatment area and then put a thin cotton towel over the area. Next place the warming pack (without the heating pad) on the area and cover yourself with a blanket. Move the pack slightly every 2 to 5 minutes. If it gets too hot, remove or add another layer in between the pack and the towel.

## Lumbago-Easing Capsules

**½ ounce turmeric root powder**  **¼ ounce Jamaican dogwood bark powder**
**½ ounce frankincense resin powder**  **¼ ounce valerian root powder**
**½ ounce yucca root powder**

Mix the powdered herbs in a bowl and fill 200 empty capsules. Take 2 capsules 2 or 3 times a day.

# ☰ MUSCLE PAIN ☰

Muscle pain can come from an injury old or new, overexertion, or generalized inflammation. One pearl of wisdom that age has taught me: when you injure yourself, don't ignore it. You must be diligent and treat it thoroughly to avoid chronic pain down the road. If you have children, teach this to them when they are young and feel indestructible. I've had many patients whose chronic pain is the result of a teenage injury that was never cared for properly.

## Topical Muscle Balm

4 ounces previously prepared
 poplar bud infused oil

2 ounces previously prepared
 arnica flower infused oil

1 tablespoon fresh hop strobiles

¼ teaspoon fresh ginger root

¼ cup olive oil

1 ounce beeswax

Put the hops and ginger in a tiny glass baking dish and add olive oil to cover. Bake at 170 degrees F for 4 hours. Allow to cool and then strain. Pour this oil along with the poplar and arnica oils into a saucepan and add the beeswax. Gently heat until the beeswax is melted. Pour into container of your choice and allow to cool. Rub into sore muscles as needed.

## Muscle-Strain Capsules

1 ounce turmeric root powder

½ ounce white willow bark powder

¼ ounce rosemary leaf powder

¼ ounce mullein leaf powder

¼ teaspoon wormwood leaf powder

Mix the powdered herbs in a bowl and fill 200 empty capsules. Take 2 capsules twice a day.

## Herbal Muscle Liniment

1 ¾ ounces myrrh resin

1 ounce comfrey leaf

1 ounce black cohosh root

1 teaspoon menthol crystals

½ teaspoon cayenne powder

16 ounces witch hazel extract

Place the ingredients in a 1-pint jar and fill to the top with witch hazel extract. Close and shake gently. Let steep for 8 weeks, gently shaking daily. Strain and transfer into container of your choice. A spray bottle is helpful to spray onto the affected area, but using a cotton pad for application works too. The idea is to create heat in the area to move the stagnated blood causing the pain.

# ≡ NEURALGIA/NEUROPATHY ≡

Neuralgia is a nerve condition where sharp shooting pains travel along the nerve track. Neuropathy is numbness and tingling along the nerve track such as in sciatica. I saw neuropathy often when I did my oncology internship in school, as chemotherapy and radiation seem to often result in nerve complaints. Imagine the sensation of hitting your funny bone over and over, or reaching to grab something and not feeling it in your hand—that is what many of my patients felt perpetually. Nerve rehabilitation became necessary, and I often used herbs that work on the nervous system.

## Painful-Nerve Tincture

2 teaspoons prickly ash bark

1 teaspoon St. John's wort leaf and flower

1 teaspoon chamomile flower

½ teaspoon oatstraw

½ teaspoon skullcap leaf

2 ounces vodka

Put the herbs in a 2-ounce jar and add vodka to fill. Close tightly and shake well. Keep in a pantry or cupboard for 3 weeks, shaking every day. Strain and transfer to a 2-ounce dropper bottle. Take 1 dropperful 3 times a day for 8 to 12 weeks.

## Nerve-Numbness Tincture

1 teaspoon prickly ash bark

1 teaspoon vervain leaf

1 teaspoon St. John's wort leaf and flower

1 teaspoon nettle leaf

2 ounces vodka

Put the herbs in a 2-ounce jar and add vodka to fill. Close tightly and shake well. Keep in a pantry or cupboard for 3 weeks, shaking every day. Strain and transfer to a 2-ounce dropper bottle. Take 1 dropperful 3 times a day for 8 to 12 weeks.

## Topical Oil for Nerve Support

4 ounces previously prepared
  St. John's wort infused oil

20 drops chamomile essential oil

10 drops marjoram essential oil

6 drops spruce essential oil

4 drops black pepper essential oil

In a 4-ounce amber bottle, add the essential oils to the St. John's wort oil. Gently massage into affected area 2 to 3 times a day.

# ≡ PERSPIRATION ≡

While perspiration is a natural bodily function, if it is absent, excessive, or extremely strong in odor, your body could be sending you a message about what's happening on the inside.

## Strong Odor Quelling Tea

*Sometimes strong odor from perspiration can signal detoxification insufficiency. A sluggish liver or digestive system can cause this, as well as skin bacteria. Supporting elimination pathways is a good place to begin.*

1¾ ounces yellow dock root

1 ounce dandelion root

1 ounce burdock root

¼ ounce licorice root

Mix the herbs in a bowl and store in a glass jar. Make tea by the cup. Simmer 1 or 2 teaspoons in 10 ounces of hot water, covered, for 10 minutes. Drink 1 to 3 cups a day for 4 to 8 weeks.

# Excessive-Perspiration Tincture

*Some folks' internal furnace runs hot or contains too much heat. The need to balance the hot and cold properties of the body is apparent. Too much sweating can lead to depletion and loss of vital fluids. This formula is also good to address high fevers that are causing excessive sweating. Some sweating during a fever is good, but too much can weaken the patient.*

2 teaspoons sage leaf

1 teaspoon schisandra berry

1 teaspoon chickweed leaf

¼ teaspoon valerian root

2 ounces vodka

Put the herbs in a 2-ounce jar and add vodka to fill. Close tightly and shake well. Keep in a pantry or cupboard for 3 weeks, shaking every day. Strain and transfer to a 2-ounce dropper bottle. Take 1 dropperful 3 times a day for 8 to 12 weeks.

# Gentle-Perspiration Tea

*Use this tea to induce gentle perspiration when you are experiencing a high fever without perspiration on the skin. It will open up the pores to free the heat.*

2 ounces lemon balm leaf

1 ounce chamomile flower

1 ounce elderflower

1 ounce yarrow leaf and flower

Mix the herbs in a bowl and store in a glass jar. Make tea by the cup. Steep 1 or 2 teaspoons in 10 ounces of hot water, covered, for 10 minutes. Try to drink the entire cup within 30 minutes.

## ═ POISON OAK/IVY ═

Leaves of three, let it be. Miraculously, I've never experienced a reaction to poison oak, but I've seen it plenty. These plants are abundant in certain regions of the United States, and if you are an avid outdoorsperson you likely know how to identify them. If you don't and if you brush against the leaves, the oil quickly penetrates the skin and can cause a rash that itches like crazy and creates blisters. Note it is the oil that is the problem, and that is why it's important to know the following to treat it. First, don't use

129

hot water to try to wash the oil off; the heat will cause the oil to spread. Do wash with bar soap and tepid water often throughout the day to contain the oil. Second, don't use oils, lotions, or salves to treat, as these oil-based products also encourage the oil of the plant to spread. Third, change the bedsheets and your clothes daily and throw directly into the washer to reduce the chance of spreading the oil to another person, or worse yet, to another area of your body.

## Poison Oak/Ivy Soothing Liniment

½ ounce white oak bark

½ ounce mugwort leaf

¼ ounce sage leaf

¼ ounce burdock root

witch hazel extract

Put the herbs in a 1-pint jar and add witch hazel extract to fill. Close tightly and shake well. Keep in a cupboard or pantry for 3 weeks, shaking every day. Strain and transfer the liquid to a clean bottle. To use, douse a cotton ball or pad with the liniment and apply to the affected area 3 times a day.

## Poison Oak/Ivy Calming Tincture

2 teaspoons chickweed leaf

1 teaspoon burdock root

1 teaspoon white willow bark

½ teaspoon black walnut hull

½ teaspoon lady's mantle

2 ounces vodka or apple cider vinegar

Put the herbs in a 2-ounce jar and add vodka or apple cider vinegar to fill. Close tightly and shake well. Keep in a pantry or cupboard for 3 weeks, shaking every day. Strain and transfer to a 2-ounce dropper bottle. Take 2 dropperfuls every 4 hours until symptoms subside.

## ⟹ SCIATICA ⟸

See "Neuralgia/Neuropathy."

# ≡ SPRAINS AND STRAINS ≡

Accidents happen. Whether it's a twisted ankle or a jammed finger, sprains and strains are a part of daily life. Some of us have a hard time determining where the limits are while exercising and tend to tip toward slightly straining our muscles. Until recently, I repeatedly overdid it. Now I look at that 50-pound bag of dog food and accept the help from the counter person offering to take it to my car for me.

## Fomentation for Sprains and Strains

1 ounce witch hazel bark

1 ounce St. John's wort leaf and flower

1 ounce comfrey leaf

1 ounce gotu kola leaf

40 drops eucalyptus essential oil

Mix the herbs in a bowl and store in a glass jar. When needed, put 6 tablespoon in a quart jar and pour boiling water over the herbs to fill the jar. Let steep 1 or 2 hours or overnight and then strain. You can keep the herbs to reuse. Warm the brew, add the essential oil, and either pour it into a bowl and soak the affected area or soak a cotton cloth and wrap the area. Treat for 20 to 30 minutes once or twice daily for temporary relief.

## Trauma Salve

1 tablespoon eucalyptus leaf

1 tablespoon gotu kola leaf

1 teaspoon rosemary leaf

½ cup olive oil

¼ cup previously prepared
  arnica infused oil

¼ cup previously prepared
  poplar bud infused oil

1 ounce beeswax

40 drops chamomile essential oil

20 drops cypress essential oil

Put the eucalyptus, gotu kola, and rosemary in a glass baking dish and add olive oil to cover. Bake at 170 degrees F for 4 hours. Allow to cool and then strain. Put all the oils into a saucepan and add the beeswax. Gently heat until the beeswax is melted. Add the essential oils and pour into container of your choice. Gently massage into the affected area 2 or 3 times a day.

# ≡ STOMACH ULCERS ≡

There are typically two types of stomach ulcers: duodenal and gastric. A duodenal ulcer is in the duodenum, where the stomach and the small intestine connect and where digestive enzymes prepare food for the next phase of digestion. A gastric ulcer is in the lining of the stomach itself. It is thought that bacteria such as *Helicobacter pylori* are a major cause of ulcers. The bacteria embed inside the lining of the stomach and duodenum, causing loss of the continuous integrity of the lining. The "holes" they create are then irritated by naturally produced digestive enzymes and stomach acid. The problem is that both of these are necessary for proper digestive function. To reduce their secretion creates a cascade of problems down the road. The principle in treating ulcers is to rid the body of harmful bacteria and heal the lining. Another contributing factor is the repetitive use of digestive-lining-damaging nonsteroidal anti-inflammatory drugs or NSAIDS, over-the-counter headache and pain medications such as acetaminophen, ibuprofen, and aspirin.

## Ulcer-Soothing Tea

2 ounces slippery elm bark

1 ounce goldenseal root

½ ounce marshmallow root

½ ounce licorice root

Mix the herbs in a bowl and store in a glass jar. Make tea by the quart. Steep 4 tablespoons in a quart jar overnight. Drink 4 6-ounce cups a day for 4 to 6 weeks.

## Ulcer-Soothing Tincture

1 teaspoon goldenseal root

1 teaspoon Oregon grape root

1 teaspoon marshmallow root

1 teaspoon yarrow flower

¼ teaspoon cinnamon bark

2 ounces vodka

Put the herbs in a 2-ounce jar and add vodka to fill. Close tightly and shake well. Keep in a pantry or cupboard for 3 weeks, shaking every day. Strain and transfer to a 2-ounce dropper bottle. Take 1 dropperful 3 times a day for 8 to 12 weeks.

## Castor Oil Pack for Ulcers

1 cup castor oil

40 drops carrot essential oil

10 drops lemongrass essential oil

5 drops frankincense essential oil

Blend the oils and apply to the abdomen. Place a thin cotton towel over the area and then a heating pad or hot water bottle. Leave on for 30 minutes every day.

## ≡ STYES ≡

Your eyes have many little glands, particularly around the eyelashes, and at times they can get blocked or clogged. This leads to irritation, and a stye can form. This looks like a little red bump on the outside of the eye and can be tender and swollen. Start with a little castor oil on the eyelid overnight and then use one of these recipes in the morning.

## Stye-Drawing Herbal Plaster

½ cup bentonite clay

¼ ounce plantain powder

¼ ounce lavender powder

Mix and store in a glass jar until needed. Blend 1/4 teaspoon with a touch of hot water and mix well. Spread over the stye and then apply a hot cloth. Keep the heat consistent on the plaster for 20 minutes.

## Stye-Relief Tincture

2 teaspoons comfrey leaf

1 teaspoon plantain leaf

1 teaspoon chickweed leaf

2 ounces vodka

Put the herbs in a 2-ounce jar and add vodka to fill. Close tightly and shake well. Keep in a pantry or cupboard for 3 weeks, shaking every day. Strain and transfer to a 2-ounce brush top bottle. Brush the tincture over the eye and allow to dry, 3 to 4 times a day.

We all have those days when we either forget the sunscreen or run out into the great outdoors after a month of winter, completely forgetting the power of the sun to scorch our winter-white skin. Herbs can heal the dermal layer and relieve the inflammation.

## Topical Sunburn-Healing Oil

1 ounce lavender flower

more lavender

oh, and don't forget the lavender

2 cups grapeseed oil

50 drops lavender essential oil

Put the lavender in a glass baking dish and cover with grapeseed oil to a depth of 1 or 2 inches. Bake at 170 degrees F for 4 hours. Allow to cool and then strain. Add the essential oil and gently mix. Apply twice daily to sunburn.

## Essential Oil Blend to Heal Sunburn

10 drops chamomile essential oil

5 drops eucalyptus radiata essential oil

5 drops lavender essential oil

2 ounces jojoba oil

Combine the oils in a 2-ounce amber bottle, mix, and store until needed. Apply to skin as needed.

## Sunburn-Healing Tincture

1 teaspoon lavender flowers

1 teaspoon comfrey leaf

1 teaspoon chickweed leaf

½ teaspoon elderflower

½ teaspoon alfalfa leaf

2 ounces vodka or apple cider vinegar

Put the herbs in a 2-ounce jar and add vodka or apple cider vinegar to fill. Close tightly and shake well. Keep in a pantry or cupboard for 3 weeks, shaking every day. Strain and transfer to a 2-ounce dropper bottle. Take 1 dropperful 3 times a day for 7 days.

# ≡ TOOTH CONDITIONS ≡

Taking care of your teeth has been proven over and over to have far-reaching benefits. The newest research shows a possible correlation between tooth and gum disease and Alzheimer's. Throughout our life, tooth pain can arise, and there are few pains more uncomfortable.

## Tincture for Loose Teeth

1 teaspoon goldenrod leaf

1 teaspoon white oak bark

1 teaspoon turmeric root

1 teaspoon birch bark

2 ounces vodka or apple cider vinegar

Put the herbs in a 2-ounce jar and add vodka or apple cider vinegar to fill. Close tightly and shake well. Keep in a pantry or cupboard for 3 weeks, shaking every day. Strain and transfer to a 2-ounce dropper bottle. Take 1 dropperful 3 times a day.

## Toothache Oil

2 teaspoons white oak bark

1 teaspoon whole cloves

1 teaspoon Jamaican dogwood bark

1 cup olive oil

5–8 drops clove essential oil

Put the herbs in a glass baking dish and cover with olive oil to a depth of 1 or 2 inches. Bake at 170 degrees F for 4 hours. Allow to cool and then strain. Add the clove essential oil and gently mix. Dip a Q-tip into the oil and rub onto the tooth and surrounding gum.

## TRADITIONAL TOOTHACHE REMEDY

A traditionally used remedy for toothache was to soak rose petals in red wine for 4 to 6 weeks and then strain. Taken in 1-ounce doses, the wine can help dull the ache. Maybe it's the rose petals or maybe it's the alcohol, but anything is worth a try with tooth pain.

## Powder for Infected Tooth

½ ounce goldenseal root powder

¼ ounce myrrh powder

¼ ounce echinacea root powder

Mix the powders and keep in a 1-ounce glass jar until needed. Moisten a Q-tip and dip it into the powder. Place the powder directly on the tooth, doing your best to allow it to seep in before saliva whisks it away. Apply 3 to 4 times a day.

## ≡ THRUSH ≡

Thrush is a normal bodily fungas, *Candida albicans*, growing in excess in the mouth and throat. Thrush can cause swelling and pain and is usually seen as a thick white fur on the tongue and in the throat areas.

## Oral Rinse for Thrush

1 ounce cranebill root

1 ounce goldenseal root

½ ounce usnea, cut up into small pieces

½ ounce echinacea root

Mix the herbs in a bowl and store in a glass jar. Steep 4 tablespoons in a pint of hot water overnight. Strain in the morning and rinse with 2 ounces 4 times a day.

## Thrush-Quell Capsules

1 ounce pau d'arco powder

¼ ounce goldenseal root powder

¼ ounce olive leaf powder

¼ ounce yarrow leaf and flower powder

¼ ounce rosehips powder

Mix the powdered herbs in a bowl and fill 200 empty capsules. Take 2 capsules 3 times a day.

## Thrush-Quell Throat Spray

3 teaspoons apple cider vinegar

15 milliliters olive leaf tincture

10 milliliters Oregon grape root tincture

10 milliliters comfrey leaf tincture

10 milliliters marshmallow root tincture

2 teaspoons distilled water

12 drops tea tree essential oil

Mix the ingredients in a 2-ounce spray bottle. Gently shake. Spray into the mouth and onto the back of the throat several times a day.

# ⇒ VARICOSE VEINS ⇐

Varicose veins range from small swollen vessels to large, painful, contorted ones. Genetics tend to play a big part in who ends up with varicose veins, but you're at risk anytime excess weight is pushing down on the lower limbs. Prolonged sitting is another contributing factor. Exercise is helpful in moving the blood. Whenever you use creams or lotions for varicose veins, always apply from the farthest point and move toward the heart. For example, start at the feet and move up the leg, in alignment with the valves of the vessels.

## Vein-Shrinking Capsules

½ ounce horse chestnut powder

½ ounce butcher's broom powder

½ ounce white oak bark powder

½ ounce yarrow powder

¼ teaspoon cayenne powder

Mix the powdered herbs in a bowl and, using gloves, fill 200 empty capsules. Take 2 capsules twice per day.

## Vein-Shrinking Topical Oil

¼ ounce butcher's broom rhizome

¼ ounce horse chestnut

¼ ounce white oak bark

¼ ounce bilberry fruit

1½ cups olive oil

15 drops cypress essential oil

10 drops tangerine essential oil

5 drops frankincense essential oil

Put the herbs in a glass baking dish and cover with olive oil to a depth of 1 or 2 inches. Bake at 170 degrees F for 4 hours. Allow to cool and then strain. Add essential oils and mix. Transfer to container of your choice and apply nightly.

## ≡ VOMITING ≡

Sometimes vomiting is necessary to protect the body. Other times, it pushes us to exhaustion, and we need to calm the purging reflex to move on to the next phase of healing. Tinctures are best for this, as teas and capsules often come right back up in the next round of vomiting. That being said, if you can get an activated charcoal capsule down, it usually helps. My go-to? Jello. I know it's strange and completely unnatural, but the sugar and gelatin often calm my stomach when vomiting cannot be controlled.

## Vomit-Quell Tincture

*If the vomiting reflex has done its job and now needs to be calmed, this tincture is indicated.*

2 teaspoons catnip leaf

½ teaspoon chamomile flower

¼ teaspoon whole cloves

¼ teaspoon lavender flower

2 ounces vodka

Put the herbs in a 2-ounce jar and add vodka to fill. Close tightly and shake well. Keep in a pantry or cupboard for 3 weeks, shaking every day. Strain and transfer to a 2-ounce dropper bottle. Take 1 dropperful every 30 minutes until symptoms subside.

## Vomit-Quell Belly Oil

¼ ounce catnip leaf

¼ ounce agrimony leaf

olive oil

20 drops chamomile essential oil

5 drops cardamom essential oil

Put the herbs in a glass baking dish and cover with olive oil to a depth of 1 or 2 inches. Bake at 170 degrees F for 4 hours. Allow to cool and then strain. Add essential oils and mix. Apply to the entire belly 3 times a day for soothing relief.

## ≡ WARTS ≡

Warts are known to be caused by the human papilloma virus, which is a lot easier to come into contact with than you may believe. The virus can enter from the tiniest of scratches on the body, even a hangnail. The immune system plays a role as well. If stress is up or your immune system is compromised, you may be more susceptible to the virus.

## Wart-B-Gone Topical Oil

¼ ounce cedar leaf

¼ ounce turmeric root

¼ ounce witch hazel bark

1 cup olive oil

20 drops cedarwood essential oil

5 drops lemon myrtle essential oil

Put the herbs in a glass baking dish and cover with olive oil to a depth of 1 or 2 inches. Bake at 170 degrees F for 4 hours. Allow to cool and then strain. Add essential oils and mix. Apply with a Q-tip 3 times a day.

## Support-Against-Warts Tea

2 ounces lemon balm leaf

1 ounce elderberry

½ ounce echinacea root

½ ounce slippery elm bark

Mix the herbs in a bowl and store in a glass jar. Make tea by the cup. Steep 1 or 2 teaspoons in 10 ounces of hot water, covered, for 10 minutes. Or make by the quart, 4 to 5 tablespoons per quart. Drink 3 cups a day.

# Immune Defense

"Sometimes the most important thing in a whole day is the rest we take between two deep breaths."

ETTY HILLESUM

IN AN AGE OF ANTIBIOTIC OVERUSE and resistance, herbs offer our bodies support when faced with run-of-the-mill colds, flus, and foreign invasions. Antibiotics are best used to combat bacterial infections and are ineffective in treating viruses, yet they are often prescribed for the latter. Bacteria and viruses have figured out new ways to shift their DNA to overcome antibiotics, which can prove a challenge to those faced with serious illness. One of the best things we can do is to reacquaint ourselves with the herbal ways. Traditionally, yarrow is known to break fevers, boneset to ease the ache of the flu, and sage to relieve a sore throat. The simple remedies of days long past offer an abundance of ways to care for ourselves and to relieve suffering.

As an herbalist for more than twenty-five years, I sometimes waver in my daily practice of using herbs, but one area where I don't waiver is my self-care when I'm sick. As a motivated, creative go-getter type, I despise being sick. It's not something I can ignore or do my best just to get through. Heck no! I attack whatever is attacking me, and I would suggest that you do the same. At the first sign of something coming on, do something about it. Drink Immune-Boost Tea, take Bug-Defense Capsules, rub oils on your chest and neck. There are plenty of approaches to choose from, but be proactive. If you notice your coworker coughing all over the place, protect yourself with a few drops of Guard's-Up Tincture. If you're getting ready to travel, dose up before getting on an airplane because once the door is shut we are all susceptible to whatever has come onboard. Same with the commuter train. Rubbing a few drops of rosemary or lavender essential oil onto your hands and chest help to block anything floating around.

A quick word about dehydration. When you're sick, sometimes it's hard enough just to lie in bed, let alone ensure you're drinking enough fluids. But upping your fluid intake is very important, especially if vomiting and/or diarrhea are present. Dehydration sneaks up on people, and before they know it they're feeling worse than they did before. When dehydration sets in, you often feel extreme fatigue accompanied by any of the following: headache, dizziness, fever and chills, nausea, muscle cramps, and/or increased heart rate. Besides keeping you hydrated, upping your fluid intake breaks up excessive mucus, prevents constipation, reduces headaches, flushes the body of toxins, and keeps blood pressure normalized. If you've been vomiting and can't keep fluids down, taking sips of Replenish Herbal Tea every 15 minutes will help calm the stomach and open up the digestive process once again.

When you fall ill, I beg you to take gentle care of yourself. If you are alone, call a friend or a delivery service to bring you items you need. Let your partner, parent, or neighbor help you. They don't need to see you in your robe, all a mess. Things like herbs and soup can be left at the door. You can thank them personally later. Our society is so bad at asking for help, yet all most of us want is to care and be cared for.

## DR. JJ'S TIPS FOR WHEN YOU FALL ILL

- Skip work, school, and events. You need to rest and have a responsibility to not expose others to your illness.

- At the onset of a cold or flu, take echinacea tincture, 1 dropperful every 3 hours for 1 or 2 days.

- Rest. I cannot overstate the value of rest when sick. Allowing the body to shut down and take care of what is ailing it makes a big difference. This doesn't mean staying home from work and being on the computer all day. It means lying in bed and trying to sleep as much as possible.

- Try a castor oil pack. The simple nature cure of a castor oil pack can mobilize the immune system to fight infection. Rub 2 tablespoons castor oil over the abdomen. Cover with a cotton towel and then a hot water bottle or heating pad. Relax for 30 to 45 minutes, or put on before bed and go to sleep.

# = ANTIVIRAL TREATMENTS =

Is it a bacteria or a virus? Generally, viruses come on slowly, create low fevers, and cause lingering symptoms, while bacterial infections come on more quickly, create higher fevers, and cause stronger first symptoms. The common cold, the flu, and a generalized sore throat are most often viral, whereas bronchitis, ear infections, strep throat, and whooping cough are most often bacterial. Bacterial infections often debilitate us. There is often no hiding the fact that we are sick. This typically forces us to cease daily routines and rest. Viral infections, on the other hand, can go on and on. This compromises the immune system, making it vulnerable to the next cold that comes along. Have you ever had one cold and been almost over it only to fall ill again? Although the symptoms of viral colds are often tolerable, we should still be aware that our body is weakened. Continuing on with our regular routine can further compromise the healing process and our health. Reach for an herbal remedy the next time a virus comes on.

## Antiviral Tea

*Whether you're up against the latest viral cold on the block or a reacquaintance with a cold sore or shingles, this tea can help you fight it off.*

2 ounces lemon balm leaf

1 ounce elderberry

¼ ounce lomatium root

¼ ounce usnea

¼ ounce yarrow flower

¼ ounce ginger root

Mix the herbs in a bowl and store in a glass jar. Steep 4 to 5 tablespoons in a quart jar and drink 3 cups a day.

# Antiviral Tincture

*Sometimes bypassing the digestive system is necessary when sick. Having direct entry through tissues can give more support to the nerves as well.*

2 tablespoons echinacea root

2 tablespoons lomatium root

1 tablespoon goldenseal root

1 tablespoon usnea

1 tablespoon licorice root

1 pint vodka

Put the herbs in a 1-pint glass jar and fill to the top with vodka. Close the lid tightly and shake well. Store in a cupboard or pantry for 3 weeks, shaking daily. Strain and transfer to container of your choice. Take 1 dropperful twice daily if experiencing high stress, or take 2 dropperfuls 3 to 4 times a day during an acute viral infection. Do not use long term.


# Antiviral Cream

*This formula is based on one originally created by herbalist Kerry Bone. I used to make it often for patients and always had positive results. Typically used for a herpes outbreak, it may also be helpful for shingles and the irritation of measles and chicken pox.*

4 ounces previously prepared
   lemon balm tincture

1 ounce St. John's wort leaf and flower

1 ounce lomatium root

4 cups water

8 ounces cocoa butter

8 ounces shea butter

2 ounces beeswax

Simmer the lemon balm tincture on the stove top on low until it is reduced by half. In a separate pan, combine the St. John's wort, the lomatium, and the water. Simmer covered on low until reduced by half and then strain. Add the reduced lemon balm tincture to the St. John's wort / lomatium extract and allow to cool slightly. In the meantime, melt the oils together in a separate pan over low heat. Once they are the same temperature, mix the extract into the oils until they emulsify and transfer to container of your choice. Apply this cream at the first tingle of a herpes outbreak and thereafter several times a day. Always use a clean Q-tip and never double dip.

# ≡ BRONCHITIS ≡

The hacking of bronchitis is distinct and hard to miss. Bronchitis can start as a cold that then drops down into the chest and settles, or it can start as a respiratory infection right off the bat. Whichever, the end result is inflammation and irritation of the lining of the bronchial tubes, which bring air into the lungs. Each time you breathe in, the lining is irritated and coughing ensues. Smokers and those whose respiratory systems are compromised are the most vulnerable. Bronchitis often leaves one feeling wiped out, with symptoms of shortness of breath, a rattling or dry cough, phlegm production, and wheezing, and upper respiratory symptoms can be present at the same time. Although typically bacterial, the cough can last for weeks as the respiratory system works to decrease the inflammation and heal from the infection.

## Acute-Bronchitis Tincture

2 teaspoons elecampane root

½ teaspoon myrrh resin

½ teaspoon cinnamon bark

½ teaspoon mullein leaf

½ teaspoon safflower flower

2 ounces vodka

Put the herbs in a 2-ounce jar and add vodka to fill. Close tightly and shake well. Keep in a pantry or cupboard for 3 weeks, shaking every day. Strain and transfer to a 2-ounce dropper bottle. Take 2 dropperfuls 3 to 4 times a day for 2 weeks.

## Bronchitis-Soothing Syrup

1 ounce elecampane root

½ ounce borage leaf

¼ ounce coltsfoot leaf

¼ ounce cinnamon bark

8 cups water

3 cups cane sugar or honey

¼ cup apple cider vinegar

Put the herbs in a saucepan with the water. Bring to a boil and reduce by half over medium-low heat. Strain the herbs out and put the brew back into the pan. Add sugar or honey and gently heat to mix if necessary, stirring continuously. Turn off the heat, add the apple cider vinegar, and allow to cool. Transfer to container of your choice and store in the refrigerator. Take 1 teaspoon 3 to 4 times a day.

# Bronchitis-Calming Tea

1 ounce peppermint leaf

¾ ounce hyssop leaf

¾ ounce elecampane root

½ ounce thyme leaf

½ ounce marshmallow root

¼ ounce sage leaf

¼ ounce vervain leaf

Mix the herbs in a bowl and store in a glass jar. Simmer 3 tablespoons over low heat in 20 ounces of water, covered, for 10 minutes. Turn off the heat, add 2 teaspoons, cover, allow to steep for 10 minutes, and then strain. You should have 18 ounces, which you can divide into 3 cups of 6 ounces each. Drink hot. When suffering from acute symptoms, drink 2 to 4 cups a day.

## ≡ CATARRH ≡

*Catarrh* is the medical term for the presence of excessive mucus or phlegm in the nose and throat. Inflammation of the mucous membranes is also present. Sometimes our nose turns into a leaky faucet with no other symptoms present. Other times we are so congested with a cold that breathing through our nose is next to impossible. Catarrh can also lead to a cough as the phlegm slides down the back of the throat and irritates the mucous membranes. Breaking up the phlegm, drawing it out, and soothing inflammation are what these herbs do best. Stay overly hydrated during these times as it helps to dilute the mucus.

# Open-Up Tincture

*Great for when excessive mucus has you blocked in your head or chest.*

2 teaspoons myrrh resin

1 teaspoon sumac bark

½ teaspoon angelica root

½ teaspoon goldenseal root

2 ounces vodka

Put the herbs in a 2-ounce jar and add vodka to fill. Close tightly and shake well. Keep in a pantry or cupboard for 3 weeks, shaking every day. Strain and transfer to a 2-ounce dropper bottle. Take 1 dropperful 3 times a day until symptoms subside.

## Catarrh-Dispersing Tea

1¼ ounces peppermint leaf

1 ounce bayberry

1 ounce coltsfoot leaf

½ ounce comfrey leaf

¼ ounce ginger root

Mix the herbs in a bowl and store in a glass jar. Make tea by the cup. Steep 1 or 2 teaspoons in 10 ounces of hot water, covered, for 10 minutes. Drink hot, 4 cups a day until symptoms subside.

## Diffuser Blend for Catarrh

5 milliliters spikenard essential oil

3 milliliters cedarwood essential oil

2 milliliters benzoin essential oil

Mix the oils in a 10-milliliter essential oil bottle. Add 5 drops to your diffuser at bedtime.

## ≡ CHEST COLDS ≡

Chest colds range from simple respiratory congestion to severe compromise. Symptoms often include cough, wheezing, sore throat, runny nose, phlegm production, tight chest, fever, and fatigue. Whenever your primary breathing system is compromised, fatigue is inevitable. Chest colds can be bacterial or viral, and the cough can vary from wet to dry to sticky. You should always treat a cough, as the longer it lasts the greater opportunity it has to take a turn for the worse. See the separate "Coughs" section to get specific with your cough for best treatment.

## Chest-Cold Tea

1 ounce mullein leaf

1 ounce elecampane root

¾ ounce rosehips

½ ounce elderflower

½ ounce elderberry

¼ ounce juniper berry

Mix the herbs in a bowl and store in a glass jar. Make tea by the cup. Steep 1 or 2 teaspoons in 10 ounces of hot water, covered, for 10 minutes. You can also steep 4 to 5 tablespoons in a quart jar, and then you have a day's worth of tea ready to go. Drink hot, 4 cups a day until symptoms subside.

## Chest-Cold Tincture

1 teaspoon usnea, pulverized or cut up

1 teaspoon yarrow flower

1 teaspoon ashwagandha root

½ teaspoon white horehound leaf

½ teaspoon marshmallow root

Put the herbs in a 2-ounce jar and add vodka to fill. Close tightly and shake well. Keep in a pantry or cupboard for 3 weeks, shaking every day. Strain and transfer to a 2-ounce dropper bottle. Take 1 to 2 dropperfuls 4 times a day.

## Chest-Cold Salve

1 tablespoon hyssop leaf

1 tablespoon licorice root

1 tablespoon ginger root

1 teaspoon lobelia leaf and flower

¾ cup olive oil

½ ounce beeswax

50 drops eucalyptus citriodora essential oil

Put the herbs in a glass baking dish and cover with olive oil to a depth of 1 or 2 inches. Bake at 170 degrees F for 4 hours. Allow to cool and then strain. Pour the oil into a saucepan and add the beeswax. Gently heat until the beeswax is melted. Add the essential oil and pour into a jar. Apply to chest, neck, and upper back.

## Diffuser Blend for Chest Colds

4 milliliters juniper essential oil

4 milliliters lemon essential oil

2 milliliters clove essential oil

Mix the oils in a 10-milliliter essential oil bottle. Add 5 drops to your diffuser at bedtime.

If you seem to catch every cold that comes your way, it's best to focus on boosting your immune function for long-term support. Teachers are often prone to low immunity as stress can be high and they are surrounded by an influx of bacteria and viruses. The elderly are another susceptible group. A typical cold can quickly turn into pneumonia if not treated and monitored diligently. In general I recommend using immunity tonics every fall before cooler temperatures result in closed windows and doors, decreasing fresh air accessibility.

## Immune-Defense Mushroom Capsules

½ ounce reishi powder

½ ounce maitake powder

½ ounce lion's mane powder

½ ounce shiitake powder

Mix the powdered herbs in a bowl and fill 200 empty capsules. Take 2 once or twice a day for 3 to 4 weeks.

## Guard's-Up Tincture

3 teaspoons echinacea root

2 ounces vodka

an additional 2 teaspoons echinacea root

Put the 3 teaspoons of echinacea root in a 2-ounce jar and add vodka to fill. Close tightly and shake well. Keep in a pantry or cupboard for 3 weeks, shaking every day. Strain and add another teaspoon of echinacea root to the tincture. Again, close tightly and shake well. Keep in a pantry or cupboard for another 3 weeks. Strain and repeat one last time. You have now created a super-charged echinacea tincture. When you are heading into treacherous waters—planes or buses or trains, highly populated places, hospitals, schools, and the like—take 5 drops. At the first sign of a cold, take 5 drops 3 times a day for 2 days.

## Build-My-Defense Tea

1 ounce astragalus root

1 ounce ashwagandha root

1 ounce reishi mushroom

½ ounce angelica root

½ ounce licorice root

Mix the herbs in a bowl and store in a glass jar. Steep 4 to 5 tablespoons in a quart of water. Drink 3 cups a day for 3 to 4 weeks.

## Immune-Defense Balm

2 tablespoons rosemary leaf

1 tablespoon lavender flower

1 tablespoon lemon balm leaf

¾ cup olive oil

½ ounce beeswax

40–60 drops essential oil of your choice: frankincense, lavender, myrtle, clove, citrus, sandalwood, vetiver, or chamomile

Put the herbs in a glass baking dish and cover with olive oil to a depth of 1 or 2 inches. Bake at 170 degrees F for 4 hours. Allow to cool and then strain. Pour the oil into a saucepan and add the beeswax. Gently heat until the beeswax is melted. Add essential oils of your choice to reach your scent preference. Apply to the neck and chest each morning before leaving the house.

Coughs are never simple. Understanding what is driving them helps to pinpoint the best herbs to relieve them. I believe a two- or three-pronged approach is best with coughs—tea and tincture as well as something topical—to kick them out of the respiratory system.

## Dry-Cough Tea

1 ounce mullein leaf

1 ounce marshmallow root

1 ounce wild cherry bark

½ ounce violet leaf

½ ounce licorice root

Mix the herbs in a bowl and store in a glass jar. Steep 4 to 5 tablespoons in a quart of water. Drink 3 cups a day for 3 to 4 weeks.

## Dry-Cough Tincture

1 teaspoon mullein leaf

1 teaspoon marshmallow root

1 teaspoon wild cherry bark

½ teaspoon violet leaf

½ teaspoon licorice root

2 ounces vodka or apple cider vinegar

Put the herbs in a 2-ounce jar and add vodka or apple cider vinegar to fill. Close tightly and shake well. Keep in a pantry or cupboard for 3 weeks, shaking every day. Strain and transfer to a 2-ounce dropper bottle. Take 2 dropperfuls 4 times daily when cough is present.

## Wet-Cough Tea

1 ounce elecampane root

1 ounce rosemary leaf

1 ounce osha root

½ ounce sage root

½ ounce licorice root

Mix the herbs in a bowl and store in a glass jar. Steep 4 to 5 tablespoons in a quart of water. Drink 3 cups a day for 3 to 4 weeks.

## Wet-Cough Tincture

*Best to have this formulated at your local herb shop for you.*

20 milliliters usnea tincture

20 milliliters osha root tincture

10 milliliters rosemary leaf tincture

5 milliliters marshmallow root tincture

5 milliliters elecampane root tincture

Mix the tinctures in a 2-ounce dropper bottle. Take 2 dropperfuls 4 times daily when cough is present.

## Expectorant Tea

*When you've got phlegm and it just isn't moving, try this tea. Be sure to drink it hot to allow the volatile oils to roll off the steam as you drink.*

1 ounce elderberry

1 ounce spearmint leaf

½ ounce elderflower

½ ounce nettle leaf

½ ounce hyssop leaf and flower

½ ounce black cohosh root

Mix the herbs in a bowl and store in a glass jar. Steep 4 to 5 tablespoons in a quart of water. Drink 3 cups a day as long as needed.

## THE STEAMY SHOWER REMEDY

Taking a steamy shower usually helps relieve symptoms when the respiratory system is compromised. Add a few drops of eucalyptus or rosemary essential oils to your shower for a therapeutic effect.

# Cough-Quell Syrup

1 ounce wild cherry bark

1 ounce marshmallow root

1 ounce hyssop leaf

½ ounce mullein leaf

½ ounce yerba santa leaf

8 cups water

3 cups cane sugar or honey

¼ cup apple cider vinegar

Put the herbs in a saucepan with the water. Bring to a boil and reduce by half on a medium-low heat. Strain out the herbs and put the brew back into the pan. Add sugar or honey and gently heat to mix if necessary, stirring continuously. Turn off the heat, add the apple cider vinegar, and allow to cool. Then transfer to container of your choice and store in the refrigerator. Take 1 teaspoon as needed.

# Ditch-the-Cough Essential Oil Blend

*This oil blend can help you sleep when coughing is keeping you awake through the night.*

4 drops ravensara essential oil

2 drops eucalyptus radiata essential oil

2 drops lavender essential oil

2 drops valerian essential oil

1 drop pine essential oil

1 ounce apricot oil

Blend the oils in a 1-ounce bottle and gently shake. Apply a couple of drops to the upper back and top of the chest before bed.

# Herbal Cough Drops

*You will need a cough drop mold for this.*

1 ounce horehound leaf

1 ounce marshmallow root

1 ounce mullein leaf

½ ounce licorice root

½ ounce cinnamon chips

¾ cup honey

Mix the herbs in a bowl and store in a glass jar. Add 4 tablespoons to a pint of hot water, close, and let steep overnight. Strain in the morning and put the infusion in a saucepan. Turn the heat on low and add honey. Bring to a boil until the liquid reaches 300 degrees F, and then pour into your mold. Allow to cool and wrap each drop in waxed paper. Store in a jar in the refrigerator. Allow to dissolve in mouth as needed.

# ≡ EARACHES ≡

The typical earache is usually caused by a bacterial infection, but it can also be viral. Calming inflammation and ridding the ear of infection are the keys to treatment. Massaging the ear also helps to drain fluid if pressure is a problem. Remember, the eardrum or tympanic membrane is a protective wall. Don't stick Q-tips or anything similar into the ear, as rupture is common. Although it can heal, the tympanic membrane is an important barrier between the inside and outside structures of the ear. If you are suffering from an earache and find a bit of blood on your pillow upon waking, it is likely the tympanic membrane has ruptured, and it is advisable to see a practitioner.

## Ear Infection Calming Tincture

2 teaspoons echinacea root

1 teaspoon chamomile flower

½ teaspoon red root

½ teaspoon licorice root

2 ounces vodka or apple cider vinegar

Put the herbs in a 2-ounce jar and add vodka or apple cider vinegar to fill. Close tightly and shake well. Keep in a pantry or cupboard for 3 weeks, shaking every day. Strain and transfer to a 2-ounce dropper bottle. Take 1 or 2 dropperfuls 3 times a day as needed.

## Earache-Soothing Tea

1 ounce elderberry

1 ounce echinacea root

1 ounce lemon balm leaf

½ ounce chamomile flower

½ ounce licorice root

Mix the herbs in a bowl and store in a glass jar. Make tea by the cup. Steep 1 or 2 teaspoons in 10 ounces of hot water, covered, for 10 minutes. Drink as needed.

## Rose-Petal Earache Infusion

2 teaspoons dried rose petals
8 ounces of water

Heat the water to boiling and steep the petals for 20 minutes. Trickle the warm infusion into the ear and allow it to rest there for a few minutes.

## Mullein-Garlic Oil for Earache

*Throughout the summer, the herb mullein grows big, beautiful stalks packed with delicate yellow flowers. These flowers have long been used to soothe ear problems. When combined with garlic, you have an antibacterial force to be reckoned with. You only get the fresh flowers in the summer, so you have to make your year's supply all at once.*

fresh mullein flowers                          olive oil
fresh garlic cloves

Fill a 4-ounce jar with mullein flowers and add olive oil to the top. Fill another 4-ounce jar with garlic cloves and add olive oil to the top. Close the jars and set out in the sun for 4 weeks, shaking daily. Every couple of days, take the lids off for a few hours to allow for water evaporation. You'll need steady temperatures to make this solar infusion, 80 degrees F or higher. After both of the oils are done, strain them. Mix 1 ounce of the mullein flower oil with ½ ounce of the garlic oil. To use, warm up slightly in the palms of your hand, drop 1 or 2 drops directly into the ear, and massage the ear gently. I gently pull up, down, and back on the ear lobe and then massage behind the ear. Can be done 3 times a day.

## Earache Pain Relief Oil

1 ounce arnica-infused oil
1 ounce poplar-infused oil

Mix the oils together. Apply a little bit behind and below the ear and massage all around the exterior surface of the ear.

## Onion Poultice for Earache

*This is an old recipe I've used a lot.*

1 yellow onion
1 tablespoon olive oil

flour of your choice

Dice the onion and sauté in olive oil until translucent. Pull from the heat and add just enough flour to make a thick paste. Find an old sock that has lost its mate and stuff it with the paste. Lay this warm sock over the ear or behind the ear for pain and congestion relief.

## ≡ FEVERS ≡

By design, fevers are our body's way of making our insides inhospitable to foreign invaders. Sometimes our body struggles to mount a fever, allowing illness to bloom. Other times fevers flare too high for too long, which can lead to a debilitated state. Encouraging them to follow their natural course can be hard, particularly when the fever compromises sleep or comfort. While over-the-counter fever reducers aid our comfort level, they often create a rebound effect, which can lead to a higher fever and prolonged illness. Trust your body, find the balance you are comfortable with, and consider these recipes for support.

## Fever-Breaking Yarrow Tea

1 teaspoon yarrow flower

Steep in 10 ounces of hot water, covered, for 10 minutes. Drink hot every few hours until fever breaks. Stop if excessive sweating is occurring so as not to reach exhaustion.

## Fever-Reducer Capsules

½ ounce white willow bark
½ ounce elderflower

½ ounce holy basil leaf
½ ounce chamomile flower

Mix the powdered herbs in a bowl and fill 200 empty capsules. Take 2 every 4 hours.

# A TRICK TO ENCOURAGE A FEVER

Try drinking hot ginger or elderflower tea while taking a hot bath to encourage a fever and light perspiration.

## Fever-Tamer Tea

*This tea helps when a fever is running too high for too long.*

¾ ounce boneset leaf

½ ounce sage leaf

½ ounce white willow bark

½ ounce fenugreek seeds

½ ounce catnip leaf

¼ ounce licorice root

Mix the herbs in a bowl and store in a glass jar. Make tea by the cup. Steep 1 or 2 teaspoons in 10 ounces of hot water, covered, for 10 minutes. Drink hot every few hours until the fever breaks.

## Fever-Cooling Compress

8 ounces cold water

30 drops rosemary essential oil

10 drops peppermint essential oil

Add the essential oils to the water and stir. Quickly soak a cotton cloth in water, wring it out, and apply it to the forehead or the nape of the neck. Refresh every 30 minutes, stirring the water each time before immersing the cloth.

# ≡ HEAD COLDS ≡

A simple head cold can be combated with so many herbal and nature cure options that there is no need to let it run its course without helping your body fight it. The congestion, headache, runny nose, sore throat, and cough that come along with it can be diminished with just a cup of tea or a few doses of tincture throughout. Be sure to check out individual sections on those things for targeted recipes. Follwing are great remedies to have in your medicine chest so when the sneezing and runny nose begin, you are prepared for battle.

## Breathe-Easier Tea

*This blend includes herbs with a high volatile oil content that work great to open up the nasal passageways. Be sure to steep the blend covered, because otherwise the oils can evaporate with the steam. Best to drink this tea hot, as it'll help break up the phlegm.*

1 ounce spearmint leaf

1 ounce peppermint leaf

½ ounce boneset leaf

½ ounce yarrow leaf and flower

½ ounce elderflower

½ ounce rosehips

Mix the herbs in a bowl and store in a glass jar. Make tea by the cup. Steep 1 or 2 teaspoons in 10 ounces of hot water, covered, for 10 minutes.

## NETI POTS FOR COLD RELIEF

I am a big proponent of neti pots and encourage their regular use, particularly during allergy and cold seasons. The practice of washing out the nose and sinus cavities aids in keeping the system free of irritating particles and excessive mucus. I for one cannot sleep without breathing through my nose, and when a cold has completely blocked that ability, a neti pot can be a life saver.

## Stop-the-Drip Tincture

*When your nose is runny and you are completely blocked, it's torture. When I lean over the sink to do the dishes and my nose drips out of control, I've reached my limit with head cold symptoms. Try this formula to dry up the drip and open up the nasal passageways.*

2 teaspoons myrrh resin

1 teaspoon chaga mushroom powder

½ teaspoon goldenseal root

½ teaspoon poke root

2 ounces vodka

Put the herbs in a 2-ounce jar and add vodka to fill. Close tightly and shake well. Keep in a pantry or cupboard for 3 weeks, shaking every day. Strain and transfer to a 2-ounce dropper bottle. Take 1 to 2 dropperfuls 3 times a day until symptoms subside.

## Congestion-Breakup Capsules

1 ounce myrrh powder

¼ ounce anise seed powder

¼ ounce holy basil leaf powder

¼ ounce Oregon grape root powder

¼ ounce cayenne powder

Use gloves due to cayenne power. Mix the powdered herbs in a bowl and fill 200 empty capsules. Take 2 capsules every 3 hours as needed.

## Decongesting Herbal Steam

*This is a good treatment before work or bed to open up the upper respiratory system. If you have access to fresh herbs, use them as the volatile oils are more abundant. You can also combine fresh and dried herbs as needed, or use just the dried herbs if that is what is available to you.*

1½ ounces lemon peel

1 ounce thyme leaf

½ ounce rosemary leaf

½ ounce peppermint leaf

½ ounce eucalyptus leaf

Combine the herbs and store in a glass jar. When needed, bring 8 to 12 cups of water to a boil in a large stockpot. Turn off the heat and add a handful or two of the herbal blend. Close the lid and let steep for 5 minutes. Take the lid off to allow the steam to roll off a bit to ensure you don't burn your face. Get a bath towel and cover your head and shoulders from behind. Lean over the pot until you feel the steam and can breathe in the scent. Stay as long as comfortable, and feel free to do little stints and then take a break. Cover the pot in between to preserve the heat and volatile oils in the steam.

## Decongesting Vapor Balm

| | |
|---|---|
| 2 tablespoons eucalyptus leaf | ¾ cup olive oil |
| 1 tablespoon thyme leaf | ½ ounce beeswax |
| 1 tablespoon rosemary leaf | pine and fir essential oils |

Put the herbs in a glass baking dish and cover with olive oil to a depth of 1 or 2 inches. Bake at 170 degrees F for 4 hours. Allow to cool and then strain. Pour the oil into a saucepan and add the beeswax. Gently heat until the beeswax is melted. Pour into container of your choice and add the essential oils. Rub a bit of balm onto the neck, under the nose, and onto the chest, and inhale. Reapply as needed.

## ≡ IMMUNE BOOST ≡

These recipes are preventive and will help you stay healthy during the onslaught of wintertime colds and flus. They are not recommended for acute situations. If you are the type of person who catches every cold that comes through, consider the recipes in the section "Chronic Low Immunity."

## Immune-Boost Tea

*Drink this from time to time throughout the year to keep the immune system sharp and ready.*

| | |
|---|---|
| 1 ounce astragalus root | ½ ounce olive leaf |
| 1 ounce holy basil leaf | ½ ounce ginkgo leaf |
| ¾ ounce elderberry | ¼ ounce ginger root |

Mix the herbs in a bowl and store in a glass jar. Steep 4 or 5 tablespoons in a quart of hot water overnight. Strain and drink 3 cups a day, either occasionally or for 1 to 2 weeks at a time to support the immune system.

## Bug-Defense Capsules

½ ounce olive leaf powder

½ ounce eleuthero root powder

¼ ounce astragalus root powder

¼ ounce elecampane root powder

¼ ounce mullein leaf powder

⅛ ounce ginger root powder

⅛ ounce cinnamon bark powder

Mix the powdered herbs in a bowl and fill 200 empty capsules. Take 2 twice per day for 2 to 3 days as needed.

## Fire Cider

*Rosemary Gladstar first concocted fire cider, a spicy hot, deliciously sweet vinegar tonic, in the kitchen at the California School of Herbal Studies in the early 1980s. Fire cider has been at the center of a trademark controversy, but as Gladstar states on her website Freefirecider. com, fire cider is for everyone to use. Here is one recipe, but there are countless others out there. Get creative and customize your own blend. Use it to boost your immune system and combat colds and flus, particularly bacterial types. A shot a day keeps the doctor away.*

½ cup fresh grated ginger root

½ cup fresh grated horseradish root

1 onion, chopped

10 cloves garlic, crushed

zest and juice from 1 lemon

2 whole astragalus roots

2 sprigs fresh or dried rosemary leaf

1 tablespoon turmeric powder

¼ teaspoon cayenne powder

organic apple cider vinegar

¼ to ⅓ cup raw local honey (optional)

Place the herbs in a quart jar and cover with apple cider vinegar, leaving 1 inch of headroom at the top. Insert a piece of parchment paper under the lid to keep the vinegar from touching the metal. Shake well and store in a cool, dark place for 6 to 8 weeks, shaking gently daily. Use cheesecloth to strain out the pulp, pouring the vinegar into a clean jar. Be sure to squeeze as much of the liquid from the pulp as you can; you may want to wear gloves as it can cause skin irritation. If you want to add honey, do it now. Heating the mixture isn't a great idea as it can destroy the probiotic healing property of vinegar, but you can gently heat the honey on low if needed and then add it to the vinegar.

# ≡ INFLUENZA, A.K.A. THE FLU ≡

Flus can be bacterial or viral, but both typically take us out of the daily living game. Body aches, headache, vomiting, diarrhea, and overall malaise are what most people report. I'm always curious when a flu rages through our household. While it's obvious that we've all contracted the same illness, it tends to present itself slightly differently in each of my family members. For me, vomiting is inevitable; my husband gets excruciating back and hip pain; my son aches all over and can never get comfortable; and my daughter seems to take it in stride, setting up camp in bed but able to enjoy the extra attention and cuddles. Luckily, and knock on wood, my husband and I tag team each other when the flu shows up, taking just one of us down at a time. For treating the flu, the keys are support, finding comfort, hydration, and rest.

## Flu-Fighter Tea

*Sipping this tea throughout the day keeps hydration up and provides the body with mini shots of herbal fighting power against the invasion.*

1 ounce chamomile flower

1 ounce rosehips

1 ounce lemon balm leaf

½ ounce boneset leaf

½ ounce yarrow flower

Mix the herbs in a bowl and store in a glass jar. Make tea by the cup. Steep 1 or 2 teaspoons in 10 ounces of hot water, covered, for 10 minutes. Sip throughout the day.

## CASTOR OIL FLU TREATMENT

Apply a castor oil pack to the abdomen twice daily to stimulate immune system circulation and clear toxins from the body. This is relatively easy to do even when you are wiped out and creates a level of comfort that allows you to relax. Rub 2 tablespoons castor oil over the abdomen. Cover with a cotton towel and then a hot water bottle or heating pad. Relax for 30 to 45 minutes, or put on before bed and go to sleep.

## Flu-Fighter Capsules

½ ounce boneset leaf powder

½ ounce elderflower powder

½ ounce activated charcoal

⅛ ounce echinacea root powder

⅛ ounce California poppy powder

⅛ ounce hops powder

⅛ ounce catnip leaf powder

Mix the powdered herbs in a bowl and fill 200 empty capsules. Take 2 capsules every 3 hours until symptoms subside.

## Flu-Fighter Essential Oil Diffuser Blend

*Flu comes on? Have the diffuser on 24/7.*

5 milliliters lemon essential oil

3 milliliters lavender essential oil

2 milliliters rosemary essential oil

Blend in a 10-milliliter essential oil bottle. Drop 5 drops into the diffuser as needed.

## ≡ LARYNGITIS ≡

Laryngitis is an inflammation of the voice box that can cause hoarseness or complete loss of the voice. Treatments directly applied to the throat are important and are best coupled with internal treatment.

## Laryngitis-Soothing Gargle

1 ounce barberry root

1 ounce echinacea root

1 ounce marshmallow root

½ ounce turmeric root

½ ounce goldenseal root

¼ cup apple cider vinegar

Mix the herbs together and store in a glass jar. Steep 4 tablespoons in a pint of hot water overnight. Strain and add the apple cider vinegar. Store in the refrigerator for up to 5 days. Gargle 1 or 2 ounces several times throughout the day as needed.

# Laryngitis Lozenges

2 ounces horehound leaf

1 ounce slippery elm bark

1 ounce chamomile flower

1 ounce ginger root

¾ cup honey

Mix the herbs in a bowl and store in a glass jar. Steep 4 tablespoons in a pint of hot water overnight. Strain in the morning and put the infusion in a saucepan. Turn the heat on low and add the honey, heating until it reaches 300 degrees F. Then pour into a lozenge mold, allow to cool, and wrap each lozenge in waxed paper. Store in a jar in the refrigerator and melt one lozenge in the mouth as needed.

# Voice-Restoring Tea

1 ounce thyme leaf

1 ounce marshmallow root

½ ounce mullein leaf

½ ounce coltsfoot leaf

½ ounce licorice root

½ ounce rose petals

Mix the herbs in a bowl and store in a glass jar. Make tea by the cup. Steep 1 or 2 teaspoons in 10 ounces of hot water, covered, for 10 minutes.

# Diffuser Blend for Laryngitis

7 milliliters rosemary essential oil

2 milliliters peppermint essential oil

1 milliliter black pepper essential oil

Mix the oils in a 10-milliliter essential oil bottle. Drop 5 drops into your diffuser as needed.

# ⇒ PINK EYE (CONJUNCTIVITIS) ⇐

Pink eye is a very common and very contagious infection. It presents as redness of the eye, often accompanied by itching and weepiness. It can be caused by viruses, bacteria, irritations, or allergies. The formulas included here target bacterial conjunctivitis but will help relieve eye irritations of any kind. Keep the kiddos home from school when they have pink eye to prevent contaminating others. Frequent hand washing is important, along with disinfecting things like keyboards, remote controls, and toys.

## Pink-Eye Wash

1 ounce calendula flower

1 ounce Oregon grape root

1 ounce myrrh resin

½ ounce chamomile flower

½ ounce chickweed leaf

Mix the herbs in a bowl and store in a glass jar until needed. Steep 5 tablespoons in a pint of hot water for 2 hours or overnight. Strain and keep in the refrigerator for up to 4 days. Saturate a cotton ball for each eye and use it to drench the eye above, below, and inside. Do not reuse cotton balls or use the same one for both eyes. Dab with a hand towel afterward. Do this 4 to 6 times a day during active infection.

## Pink-Eye Tincture

*Take this tincture at the same time to fight the infection internally.*

1 teaspoon echinacea root

1 teaspoon licorice root

½ teaspoon dandelion root

½ teaspoon blackberry leaf

½ teaspoon Oregon grape root

½ teaspoon calendula flower

2 ounces vodka or apple cider vinegar

Put the herbs in a 2-ounce jar and add vodka or apple cider vinegar to fill. Close tightly and shake well. Keep in a pantry or cupboard for 3 weeks, shaking every day. Strain and transfer to a 2-ounce dropper bottle. Take 2 dropperfuls 3 times a day during acute infection.

A respiratory infection often results in a sinus infection, or for some, sinus infections just develop all on their own. I've repeatedly discovered with my chronic sinusitis patients that diet clearly plays a role, and there is often a direct correlation with sugar, gluten, and dairy intake. Committing to an anti-inflammatory diet has greatly reduced the frequency and severity of chronic or repeated sinus infections for most of my patients. Being diligent with self-care once a sinus infection is suspected can greatly reduce symptoms and discomfort.

## Sinusitis-Relief Infusion

*The age-old tradition of washing out the nasal passageways helps to clear them of sinus-causing germs. It can also increase breathing capacity and soothe the membranes of the upper respiratory tract. Several of my patients who suffered tremendously from chronic sinus infections have found relief with the use of a neti pot in the treatment plan. Even if you are completely blocked, using a neti pot can eventually break through the wall of mucus and provide sweet relief. Try using just salt first, 1 teaspoon to 16 ounces of lukewarm water. Then try this infusion.*

**1 tablespoon marshmallow root**
**1 tablespoon goldenseal root**

Steep the herbs in 8 ounces of room temperature water for 2 hours or overnight. Strain and save the herbs for reuse. For an active sinus infection, blend 1 teaspoon salt, 2 ounces of the infusion, and 12 ounces of lukewarm water and run it through the sinuses. If you suspect mold is an issue, add 1 dropperful of black walnut hull tincture to 16 ounces of lukewarm water.

## Sinus-Relief Capsules

**½ ounce hyssop leaf powder**
**½ ounce myrrh resin powder**
**½ ounce nettle leaf powder**

**¼ ounce fennel seed powder**
**⅛ ounce horseradish powder**

Mix the powdered herbs in a bowl and fill 200 empty capsules. Take 2 capsules 3 times a day until symptoms subside.

## Sinus-Relief Tea

1¼ ounces orange peel

1 ounce rosehips

½ ounce hyssop leaf

½ ounce mullein leaf

½ ounce thyme leaf

¼ ounce licorice root

Mix the herbs in a bowl and store in a glass jar. Make tea by the cup. Steep 1 or 2 teaspoons in 10 ounces of hot water, covered, for 10 minutes. Sip throughout the day.

## Sinus Balm

2 tablespoons rosemary leaf

2 tablespoons elderflower

1 tablespoon white willow bark

1 tablespoon plantain leaf

¾ cup olive oil

½ ounce beeswax

40 drops pine essential oil

15 drops geranium essential oil

5 drops benzoin essential oil

Put the herbs in a glass baking dish and cover with olive oil to a depth of 1 or 2 inches. Bake at 170 degrees F for 4 hours. Allow to cool and then strain. Pour the oil into a saucepan and add the beeswax. Gently heat until the beeswax is melted. Pour into container of your choice and add essential oils. Rub this on your forehead and nose for temporary relief of sinus pain and pressure.

## ≡ SORE THROAT ≡

My red flag that illness is hovering is a sore throat. Having suffered from chronic strep throat as a child, I know this is my susceptible point and when I feel that all-too-familiar sensation, I get on it. Most sore throats that are part of a cold are caused by viral infections, while strep throat is bacterial. Sore throats can also be caused by allergies, air contaminants, digestive issues, and smoking.

# Sore-Throat Spray

*A topical blast directly onto the tissues can help ease the pain and fight the infection.*

2 teaspoons prickly ash bark

1 teaspoon sage leaf

1 teaspoon echinacea root

½ teaspoon myrrh resin

1 ounce apple cider vinegar

1 ounce vegetable glycerin

Put the herbs in a 2-ounce jar and add apple cider vinegar and glycerin to fill. Close tightly and shake well. Keep in a pantry or cupboard for 3 weeks, shaking every day. Strain and transfer to a 2-ounce spray bottle. Spray 1 or 2 times into the mouth and toward the throat as needed.

# Throat-Soothing Tea

2 ounces sage leaf

1 ounce mullein leaf

½ ounce slippery elm bark

½ ounce licorice root

⅛ ounce whole cloves

Mix the herbs in a bowl and store in a glass jar. Make tea by the cup. Steep 1 or 2 teaspoons in 10 ounces of hot water, covered, for 10 minutes. Sip as needed throughout the day.

# Throat-Soothing Tincture

2 teaspoons sage leaf

1 teaspoon echinacea root

1 teaspoon hyssop leaf

½ teaspoon elderberry

½ teaspoon red root

2 ounces vodka or apple cider vinegar

Put the herbs in a 2-ounce jar and add vodka or apple cider vinegar to fill. Close tightly and shake well. Keep in a pantry or cupboard for 3 weeks, shaking every day. Strain and transfer to a 2-ounce dropper bottle. Take 1 or 2 dropperfuls 3 times a day.

## Sore-Throat Lozenges

2 ounces rosehips

1 ounce slippery elm bark

1 ounce marshmallow root

1 ounce prickly ash bark

¾ cup honey

80–100 drops orange essential oil

Mix the herbs in a bowl and store in a glass jar. Steep 5 tablespoons in a pint of hot water overnight. Strain in the morning and put the infusion in a saucepan. Turn the heat on low and add the honey, heating until it reaches 300 degrees F. Allow to cool slightly and add the essential oil. Then pour into a lozenge mold, allow to cool, and wrap each lozenge in waxed paper. Store in a jar in the refrigerator and melt one lozenge in the mouth as needed.

## ≡ STAPH INFECTIONS ≡

Staph infections are bacterial and typically reside on the skin, but internal staph infections such as food poisoning and toxic shock syndrome are also possible. Considered highly contagious, staph often presents on the skin in the form of a boil, a furuncle, an abscess, or a collection of pus. It can also present with a crust that looks like dried honey, typical of impetigo. Keep the area clean and disinfected to resolve the infection. Honey has been used as an effective healing agent for staph infections for centuries.

## Staph-Fighting Spray

*Use this spray to fight infection and keep the area clean.*

½ ounce lavender flower

½ ounce calendula flower

½ ounce yarrow flower

½ ounce goldenseal root

12 ounces distilled water

3 ounces apple cider vinegar

1 ounce vodka

Put the herbs in a pint jar and add the distilled water, apple cider vinegar, and vodka. Close tightly and shake well. Keep in a pantry or cupboard for 3 weeks, shaking every day. Strain and transfer to a 2-ounce spray bottle. Spray onto the affected area 4 times a day, allowing it to dry. Alternatively, you can spray a cotton pad and affix it to the area with gauze, changing the dressing 3 times a day.

## Staph-Fighting Tincture

*Best to support the body from the inside out when dealing with staph infections.*

2 teaspoons echinacea root

1 teaspoon Oregon grape root

1 teaspoon usnea, cut up finely

1 teaspoon calendula flower

2 ounces vodka or apple cider vinegar

Put the herbs in a 2-ounce jar and add vodka or apple cider vinegar to fill. Close tightly and shake well. Keep in a pantry or cupboard for 3 weeks, shaking every day. Strain and transfer to a 2-ounce dropper bottle. Take 1 or 2 dropperfuls 3 times a day.

## ≡ STREP THROAT ≡

See also "Sore Throat."
The following recipes are specific to strep throat infections.

## Strep-Relief Tea

1 ounce echinacea root

1 ounce orange peel

½ ounce osha root

½ ounce hyssop leaf

½ ounce sage leaf

½ ounce wild cherry bark

Mix the herbs in a bowl and store in a glass jar. Make tea by the cup. Steep 1 or 2 teaspoons in 10 ounces of hot water, covered, for 10 minutes. Drink 3 cups a day, sweetening with honey to taste.

## Strep-Fighting Tincture

2 teaspoons echinacea root

1 teaspoon wireweed leaf

1 teaspoon lomatium root

1 teaspoon sage leaf

2 ounces vodka or apple cider vinegar

Put the herbs in a 2-ounce jar and add vodka or apple cider vinegar to fill. Close tightly and shake well. Keep in a pantry or cupboard for 3 weeks, shaking every day. Strain and transfer to a 2-ounce dropper bottle. Take 2 dropperfuls, holding it in the mouth for 30 seconds and then allowing it to slowly slide into the throat before swallowing.

When the glands in your neck and throat area are swollen, your body is trying to tell you something. Respond with these recipes to support the lymphatic system.

## Lymph Congestion Relief Oil

2 tablespoons poke root

1 tablespoon fennel seed

½ tablespoon lobelia leaf

¾ cup olive oil

45 drops grapefruit essential oil

15 drops rosemary essential oil

Put the herbs in a glass baking dish and cover with olive oil to a depth of 1 or 2 inches. Bake at 170 degrees F for 4 hours. Allow to cool and then strain. Transfer to bottle of your choice and add the essential oils. Rub 1 teaspoon over the neck glands to help reduce swelling.

## Lymphatic-Support Capsules

¾ ounce burdock root

½ ounce figwort leaf

½ ounce violet leaf

¼ ounce stone root

Mix the powdered herbs in a bowl and fill 200 empty capsules. Take 2 capsules twice a day.

## Tea for Swollen Glands

1 ounce pipsisssewa leaf

1 ounce cleavers leaf

½ ounce white willow leaf

½ ounce calendula flower

½ ounce hibiscus fruit

½ ounce lemongrass

Mix the herbs in a bowl and store in a glass jar. Make tea by the cup. Steep 1 or 2 teaspoons in 10 ounces of hot water, covered, for 10 minutes. Drink hot, 2 to 3 cups a day for 4 to 5 days.

# Women's Health

---🌿---

"A weed is a plant whose virtue is
not yet known."

RALPH WALDO EMERSON

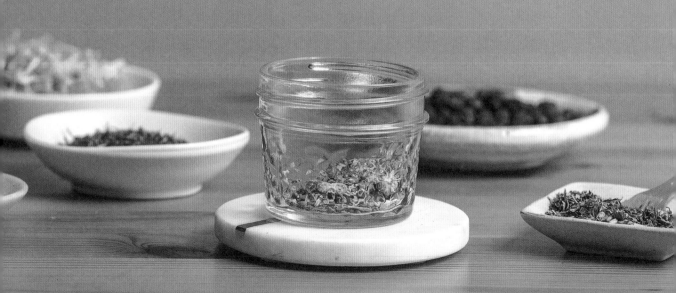

I CAN ONLY SPEAK FOR MYSELF, but I know a lot of women like me. I tend to overgive and often put others' needs, wants, and desires in front of my own. I have children that I adore, and their needs often come first. I'm in a committed marriage, I care for animals in need, I run an herb shop to fulfill others' dreams of working with herbs, and I run a household. I also have goals I want to achieve. I often find myself communing with the moon, staring up at her and asking for support, blessings, guidance, and strength, but most of all asking for balance. I ask her to show me how I can achieve all that I desire yet still have time for myself.

Women tend to take on so much that we do not have time to care for ourselves properly. When was the last time you took a walk by yourself, created art, or relaxed in the bath? If the answer is "I have no idea," it's time to carve out a little space for self-care. I encourage you to learn and use the recipes in this section as part of a larger commitment to self-care. These recipes are focused on physically supporting the female body with herbs, which are nurturing by nature and which work in profound but gentle ways.

## ABSENCE OF MENSES

The absence of menses, or amenorrhea, can be triggered by pregnancy, breastfeeding, menopause, or some methods of birth control. If you can rule these out and you have had menses at one point in your life but not now, consider the following possible causes: hormone imbalance, thyroid issues, low body weight, or stress. Once you've had a physical exam from your health care provider and have determined that your problem is hormone imbalance or stress, consider these blends for tonification and support of the reproductive system.

## Amenorrhea-Busting Capsules

½ ounce dong quai root powder

½ ounce vitex berry powder

½ ounce spirulina powder

¼ ounce kelp powder

¼ ounce licorice root powder

Mix the powdered herbs in a bowl and fill 200 empty capsules. Take 2 of these twice daily to encourage regulation of reproductive function and hormone balance.

## Reproductive-Health Tea

1½ ounces vitex berry

1 ounce black cohosh root

½ ounce wild yam root

½ ounce yellow dock root

¼ ounce licorice root

¼ ounce ginger root

Mix the herbs in a bowl and store in a glass jar. When needed, put 4 or 5 tablespoons in a quart jar and pour boiling water over the herbs to fill the jar. Let steep overnight and strain in the morning. Drink 3 cups a day for 6 to 12 weeks.

## Bring-on-the-Menses Tea

*When menses are delayed and pregnancy has been ruled out, this formula encourages the menstrual cycle to begin.*

2 ounces peppermint leaf

1½ ounces parsley leaf

¼ ounce sage leaf

¼ ounce rosemary leaf

Mix the herbs in a bowl and store in a glass jar. When needed, put 4 or 5 tablespoons in a quart jar and pour boiling water over the herbs to fill the jar. Let steep overnight and then strain. Drink 3 cups a day for 3 to 5 days, stopping once menses begin.

# ≡ BLADDER INCONTINENCE ≡

A feeling of urgency or the inability to hold urine in the absence of infection can be the result of pregnancy, age, hormonal changes, surgery, or medications. The focus of treatment is to tone up the bladder and its surrounding ligaments. If a lack of hormones due to post pregnancy, hysterectomy, or menopause is to blame, herbs can help support the reproductive hormones.

## Bladder-Toning Tincture

2 teaspoons hydrangea root

1 teaspoon agrimony leaf

1 teaspoon goldenrod leaf

1 teaspoon burdock root

1 teaspoon horsetail leaf

2 ounces vodka or apple cider vinegar

Put the herbs in a 2-ounce jar and add vodka or apple cider vinegar to fill. Close tightly and shake well. Keep in a pantry or cupboard for 3 weeks, shaking every day. Strain and transfer to a 2-ounce dropper bottle. Take 1 dropperful 3 times a day for 4 to 6 weeks.

## Incontinence-Quelling Capsules

½ ounce pipsissewa leaf

½ ounce agrimony leaf

¼ ounce catnip leaf

¼ ounce raspberry leaf

¼ ounce white oak bark

¼ ounce sumac berry

Mix the powdered herbs in a bowl and fill 200 empty vegetable capsules. Take 2 capsules twice a day for 4 to 6 weeks.

## Hormone-Support Tincture

*Using estrogenic herbs can be helpful if lack of estrogen is causing loss of bladder tone.*

2 teaspoons red clover blossoms

1 teaspoon burdock root

1 teaspoon black cohosh root

1 teaspoon agrimony leaf

1 teaspoon raspberry leaf

2 ounces vodka or apple cider vinegar

Put the herbs in a 2-ounce jar and add vodka or apple cider vinegar to fill. Close tightly and shake well. Keep in a pantry or cupboard for 3 weeks, shaking every day. Strain and transfer to a 2-ounce dropper bottle. Take 1 dropperful 3 times a day for 6 to 8 weeks.

# ≡ BLADDER INFECTIONS ≡

Cystitis, or a bladder infection, should always trigger you to consult your health care provider as the infection can quickly ascend to the kidneys and cause permanent damage. The formulas here are for support while waiting or at the first familiar sign of impending infection. Taking small doses frequently is the best approach.

## Bladder-Support Tincture

2 teaspoons goldenseal root

1 teaspoon myrrh resin

1 teaspoon uva ursi leaf

½ teaspoon slippery elm bark

½ teaspoon cornsilk

2 ounces vodka

Put the herbs in a 2-ounce jar and add vodka to fill. Close tightly and shake well. Keep in a pantry or cupboard for 3 weeks, shaking every day. Strain and transfer to a 2-ounce dropper bottle. Take 1 or 2 dropperfuls every 2 hours until symptoms subside.

## Bladder-Support Tea

1 ounce yarrow leaf and flower

1 ounce marshmallow root

½ ounce Oregon grape root

½ ounce uva ursi leaf

½ ounce dandelion leaf

½ ounce cornsilk

Mix the herbs in a bowl and store in a glass jar. When needed, put 4 or 5 tablespoons in a quart jar and pour boiling water over the herbs to fill the jar. Let steep overnight and strain in the morning. Drink 3 cups a day.

## Bladder-Support Capsules

½ ounce cranberry powder

½ ounce goldenseal root powder

½ ounce uva ursi leaf powder

¼ ounce dandelion leaf

¼ ounce pipsisssewa leaf

Mix the powdered herbs in a bowl and fill 200 empty capsules. Take 2 capsules 3 times a day.

"The sun of my smile, / The ride of my breasts, / The grace of my style. / I'm a woman," wrote Maya Angelou in her poem "Phenomenal Woman." Breasts are both a physical and an emotional aspect of being a woman. Having a relationship with your breasts is just like having a relationship with any other part of your body. Knowing the terrain and the sensations and when something isn't normal gives you insight into the health of your body. Many women have fibrocystic breasts, meaning the breast tissue feels lumpy, with the lumps being round or ropey, tender or not. As with any lymphatic tissue, breast tissue can become stagnant or congested. Just like massaging a muscle, you can massage your breasts with herbal oils to break up the fibrotic tissue.

## Breast Massage Oil

*Massaging this oil into the breasts has been proven to reduce fibrocystic breast tissue.*

2 tablespoon cleavers leaf

1 tablespoon poke root

2 teaspoons ginger root

olive oil

Put the herbs in a glass baking dish and cover with olive oil to a depth of 1 or 2 inches. Bake at 170 degrees F for 4 hours. Allow to cool and then strain. Use the oil to gently massage the breasts once a day for 5 days, 4 times a year. Alternatively, you can use once a week for 12 weeks and then take 12 weeks off.

## Breast-Health Tincture

2 teaspoons burdock root

1 teaspoon cleavers leaf

1 teaspoon astragalus root

½ teaspoon kelp

½ teaspoon motherwort leaf

2 ounces vodka or apple cider vinegar

Put the herbs in a 2-ounce jar and add vodka or apple cider vinegar to fill. Close tightly and shake well. Keep in a pantry or cupboard for 3 weeks, shaking every day. Strain and transfer to a 2-ounce dropper bottle. Take 1 dropperful twice daily for 3 weeks.

## Breast-Health Tonic Tea

1 ounce peppermint leaf

¾ ounce pau d'arco leaf

¾ ounce burdock root

½ ounce vitex berry

½ ounce cleavers leaf

¼ ounce yarrow leaf and flower

¼ ounce chamomile flower

Mix the herbs in a bowl and store in a glass jar. When needed, put 4 or 5 tablespoons in a quart jar and pour boiling water over the herbs to fill the jar. Let steep overnight and drink 3 cups a day for 8 to 12 weeks.

≡ FERTILITY ≡

When you decide you're ready to have a baby, very little can take your mind off the task. Unfortunately this thought process can lead to stress, especially if conception doesn't come as fast as you'd like. Do what you can to stay grounded and patient through the process. These recipes are to help with that as well as to support the uterus, ovaries, and hormones.

## Fertile-Ground Tea

1 ounce vitex

1 ounce rhodiola root bark

½ ounce bupleurum root

½ ounce lemongrass

¼ ounce angelica root

¼ ounce vervain

¼ ounce ginger

¼ ounce cinnamon

Mix the herbs in a bowl and store in a glass jar. When needed, put 4 or 5 tablespoons in a quart jar and pour boiling water over the herbs to fill the jar. Let steep overnight and strain in the morning. Drink 3 cups a day for 4 to 6 weeks.

# Fertility Tincture

2 teaspoons partridge berry

1 teaspoon yellow dock root

1 teaspoon milk thistle seed

1 teaspoon dong quai root

1 teaspoon vitex berry

2 ounces vodka

Put the herbs in a 2-ounce jar and add vodka to fill. Close tightly and shake well. Keep in a pantry or cupboard for 3 weeks, shaking every day. Strain and transfer to a 2-ounce dropper bottle. Take 1 dropperful 3 times a day.

# Conception-Tonic Capsules

½ ounce maca root

½ ounce schisandra berry

½ ounce skullcap leaf

¼ ounce burdock root

¼ ounce gentian root

Mix the powdered herbs in a bowl and fill 200 empty capsules. Take 2 capsules twice a day for 4 to 6 weeks.

# Castor Oil Pack for Fertility Support

¼ ounce ginger root

½ ounce vervain

¼ ounce lavender flowers

15 drops sage essential oil

10 drops ylang ylang essential oil

5 drops geranium essential oil

castor oil

Put the herbs in a glass baking dish and cover with castor oil to a depth of 1 to 2 inches. Bake at 170 degrees F for 4 hours. Allow to cool and then strain. Add essential oils and transfer to bottle of your choice. Once daily, spread 2 tablespoons of the oil blend over the abdomen. Cover with a cotton towel and then a hot water bottle or heating pad. Relax for 30 to 45 minutes, or put on before bed and go to sleep. Skip when menstruating.

Heavy bleeding, or menorrhagia, is when you are bleeding through a pad or tampon in 2 hours or less. It is advisable to see your health care practitioner if heavy bleeding is occurring with each cycle to rule out anemia and/or fibroids.

## Menorrhagia-Stop Tincture

**2 teaspoons shepherd's purse leaf**     **2 ounces vodka**
**1 teaspoon cinnamon chips**

Put the herbs in a 2-ounce jar and add vodka to fill. Close tightly and shake well. Keep in a pantry or cupboard for 3 weeks, shaking every day. Strain and transfer to a 2-ounce dropper bottle. Take 2 dropperfuls every 30 to 40 minutes to slow excessive menstrual bleeding.

## Menorrhagia-Relief Tea

**1 ounce raspberry leaf**          **½ ounce blackberry leaf**
**1 ounce shepherd's purse leaf**   **½ ounce yarrow leaf and flower**
**½ ounce sage leaf**               **½ ounce cinnamon chips**

Mix the herbs in a bowl and store in a glass jar. When needed, put 4 or 5 tablespoons in a quart jar and pour boiling water over the herbs to fill the jar. Let steep overnight and strain in the morning. Drink 3 cups a day on your heavy days.

## Menorrhagia-Relief Fomentation

**2 ounces rose petals**       **1 ounce sage leaf**
**1 ounce hawthorn flower**

Mix the herbs in a bowl and store in a glass jar. When needed put 5 tablespoons in a pint jar and pour boiling water over the herbs to fill the jar. Let steep 2 to 4 hours or overnight. Strain and soak a cotton cloth in the infusion. Place over the lower abdomen and apply gentle heat for 30 minutes.

When your menses either do not come monthly or vary greatly in length from month to month, this can be caused by hormone fluctuations, ovulation problems, some birth control methods, or stress, to name a few. Using a journal or app to keep track of your cycle can help you identify any pattern.

## Menses-Regulating Capsules

*This blend focuses on hormone balance and ovarian support.*

½ ounce dong quai root powder

½ ounce vitex berry powder

¼ ounce burdock root powder

¼ ounce spirulina powder

¼ ounce partridge berry powder

¼ ounce vervain powder

Mix the powdered herbs in a bowl and fill 200 empty capsules. Take 2 capsules twice a day.

## Menstrual-Balance Tincture

*This blend balances and tones the reproductive system.*

2 teaspoons vitex berry

1 teaspoon motherwort leaf

½ teaspoon safflower flower

½ teaspoon wild yam root

2 ounces vodka

Put the herbs in a 2-ounce jar and add vodka to fill. Close tightly and shake well. Keep in a pantry or cupboard for 3 weeks, shaking every day. Strain and put into a 2-ounce dropper bottle. Take 1 dropperful 3 times a day.

## Castor Oil Pack for Menstrual Support

2 tablespoons black cohosh root

1 tablespoon lady's mantle leaf

1 tablespoon rose petals

castor oil

Put the herbs in a glass baking dish and cover with castor oil to a depth of 1 or 2 inches. Bake at 170 degrees F for 4 hours. Allow to cool and then strain. Apply 1 or 2 tablespoons over the abdomen and cover with a cotton cloth. Apply gentle heat for 30 to 45 minutes. Ideally use packs 4 consecutive days a week for weeks 1 to 3 of the menstrual cycle.

As more mothers have returned to breastfeeding their children, more women are concerned that they're not making enough milk for their baby. Keeping stress down and focusing on what is best for baby are important. These blends are packed with herbs traditionally used to support the mother and increase breast milk supply.

## Breast Milk Supply Tea

*Hydration always helps!*

1 ounce goat's rue leaf

1 ounce fennel seed

¾ ounce nettle leaf

½ ounce blessed thistle

½ ounce skullcap leaf

¼ ounce anise seed

Mix the herbs in a bowl and store in a glass jar. When needed, put 4 or 5 tablespoons in a quart jar and pour boiling water over the herbs to fill the jar. Let steep overnight and strain in the morning. Drink 3 cups a day.

## Breast Milk Supply Capsules

½ ounce fennel seed powder

½ ounce fenugreek seed powder

¼ ounce shatavari root powder

¼ ounce blessed thistle powder

¼ ounce hops powder

¼ ounce spirulina powder

Mix the powdered herbs in a bowl and fill 200 empty capsules. Take 2 capsules 3 times a day.

## ≡ LEUCORRHEA ≡

Any discharge from the vagina that is excessive and deviates from your normal can be considered leucorrhea. First rule out a bacterial or yeast infection. Then consider the thicker discharge typical of ovulation to ensure you aren't thinking your normal is abnormal. Checking in with your health care provider can help you assess. If all of those check out, consider using astringent herbs to tone the reproductive system.

## Calm-the-Discharge Tea

| | |
|---|---|
| 1 ounce ashwagandha root | ½ ounce witch hazel leaf |
| 1 ounce blackberry leaf | ½ ounce Oregon grape root |
| ½ ounce red clover blossoms | ½ ounce hibiscus flower |

Mix the herbs in a bowl and store in a glass jar. When needed, put 4 or 5 tablespoons in a quart jar and pour boiling water over the herbs to fill the jar. Let steep overnight and strain in the morning. Drink 1 to 3 cups a day for 4 weeks.

## Leucorrhea Cordial

| | |
|---|---|
| 1 ounce green tea | ¼ ounce rosemary leaf |
| ½ ounce white oak bark | ¼ ounce ginger root |
| ½ ounce raspberry leaf | 6 whole cloves |
| ¼ ounce cardamom | 6 dried apricots |
| ¼ ounce fennel seed | 2 cups red wine or brandy |

Soak the ingredients in the wine or brandy for 8 weeks, shaking daily. Strain and transfer into bottle of your choice. Store in a cool, dark place. Take ½-ounce doses twice daily for treatment.

## Leucorrhea Salve

| | |
|---|---|
| 1 tablespoon cumin seed | 1 tablespoon ashwagandha root |
| 1 tablespoon turmeric root | ¾ cup olive oil |
| 1 tablespoon raspberry leaf | ½ ounce beeswax |

Put the herbs in a glass baking dish and cover with olive oil to a depth of 1 or 2 inches. Bake at 170 degrees F for 4 hours. Allow to cool and then strain. Pour the oil into a saucepan and add the beeswax. Gently heat until the beeswax is melted. Pour into container of your choice. Apply twice daily to the external parts of the vagina to support the health of the mucous membranes.

# ≡ MENOPAUSE ≡

Menopause actually begins twelve months before the complete cessation of menses when the hormones start shifting and preparing for a new balance and purpose. Reproduction is no longer the focus and energy is now conserved for other purposes as we age. Many women experience a sense of freedom, while others feel a sense of loss. Make room for whatever you are feeling and take the time to honor it. Symptoms such as hot flashes and insomnia often occur and can be addressed with herbs that support the transition to a new normal of hormone balance.

## Hot-Flash Cooling Tincture

2 teaspoons black cohosh root

1 teaspoon motherwort leaf

1 teaspoon sage leaf

1 teaspoon spearmint leaf

2 ounces vodka

Put the herbs in a 2-ounce jar and add vodka to fill. Close tightly and shake well. Keep in a pantry or cupboard for 3 weeks, shaking every day. Strain and transfer to a 2-ounce dropper bottle. Take 1 or 2 dropperfuls as needed.

## Menopause-Balance Capsules

½ ounce angelica root powder

½ ounce burdock root powder

½ ounce turmeric root powder

¼ ounce black cohosh root powder

¼ ounce licorice root powder

Mix the powdered herbs in a bowl and fill 200 empty capsules. Take 2 capsules twice a day.

## Menopause Sleep Support Tincture

1 teaspoon skullcap leaf

1 teaspoon wild yam root

1 teaspoon dong quai root

½ teaspoon sage leaf

½ teaspoon hop strobiles

2 ounces vodka

Put the herbs in a 2-ounce jar and add vodka to fill. Close tightly and shake well. Keep in a pantry or cupboard for 3 weeks, shaking every day. Strain and transfer to a 2-ounce dropper bottle. Take 2 dropperfuls twice daily.

# Wise-Woman Tea

*Keeping the mineral intake up during the transition to menopause supports bones and digestive function, promoting longevity of body, mind, and spirit.*

1 ounce alfalfa leaf

1 ounce nettle leaf

½ ounce comfrey leaf

½ ounce catnip leaf

¼ ounce fennel seed

¼ ounce sage leaf

¼ ounce ginger root

¼ ounce licorice root

Mix the herbs in a bowl and store in a glass jar. When needed, put 4 or 5 tablespoons in a quart jar and pour boiling water over the herbs to fill the jar. Let steep overnight and strain in the morning. Drink 1 to 3 cups a day as desired.

## ═ MENSTRUAL CRAMPING ═

In our fast-paced modern world, we women rarely stop to care for ourselves when our menses begin each month. We have school, work, kids, responsibilities, and engagements to tend to, so we need support for whatever we are experiencing. Herbs are here to help. And if you can find the space for downtime—take it.

# Cramp-Stop Tincture

1 teaspoon silk tassel leaf

2 teaspoons cramp bark

1 teaspoon California poppy
    flower and leaf

½ teaspoon black cohosh root

½ teaspoon valerian root

2 ounces vodka or apple cider vinegar

Put the herbs in a 2-ounce jar and add vodka or apple cider vinegar to fill. Close tightly and shake well. Keep in a pantry or cupboard for 3 weeks, shaking every day. Strain and transfer to a 2-ounce dropper bottle. Take 2 or 3 dropperfuls as needed, not to exceed 6 doses in 8 hours.

## Cramp-Relief Capsules

½ ounce cramp bark powder

½ ounce lemongrass powder

½ ounce skullcap leaf powder

¼ ounce hops powder

¼ ounce valerian root powder

¹⁄₁₆ ounce black pepper powder

Mix the powdered herbs in a bowl and fill 200 empty capsules. Take 2 capsules at the onset of menstrual cramping.


## Cramp-Relief Poultice

*A ginger root poultice is known to reduce menstrual cramping and is a warm and soothing treatment. You must first simmer the root to release its medicinal properties and can enjoy the fragrance as you are waiting.*

2 cups water

½ cup freshly grated ginger root

Combine the water and the root and simmer on low, covered, for 10 minutes. Strain out the ginger root and set it on a thin cotton cloth the size of a washcloth. Fold the cloth to the size of a paperback book to enclose the ginger root. Squeeze so the cloth becomes saturated and place it over the area of cramping, typically the uterus. Apply a hot water bottle or heating pad over it and relax for 15 to 20 minutes.


## PMS, EMOTIONAL ASPECTS

Many symptoms accompany premenstrual syndrome (PMS), but these recipes are to support the emotional balance aspect. Some women feel irritated, weepy, sensitive, or downright angry before their menses. While our life experiences are the instigators of what we feel, hormones are often the cause of feeling these emotions more strongly. Using herbs to tone the reproductive and nervous systems helps to balance out hormones and support a more balanced sense of self premenstrually.

# Positive-Self Capsules

*These can be taken throughout the month to promote a positive sense of self and to create balance within the endocrine system.*

½ ounce rhodiola root

½ ounce skullcap leaf

¼ ounce vitex berry

¼ ounce partridge berry

¼ ounce cramp bark

¼ ounce burdock root

Mix the powdered herbs in a bowl and fill 200 empty capsules. Take 2 capsules once or twice daily throughout the month.

# Emotional Well-Being Blend

*Flower essences work on the emotional aspects of health and healing. They come in drop form and taste like sweet water.*

7 drops cherry plum flower essence

7 drops mustard flower essence

7 drops impatiens flower essence

7 drops beech flower essence

distilled water

30 drops brandy

Mix the flower essences in a 1-ounce dropper bottle and fill almost to the top with distilled water. Add the brandy for preservation. Take 4 drops 4 times a day for as long as needed.

# Emotional Strength Tincture

1 teaspoon agrimony leaf

1 teaspoon passionflower leaf

1 teaspoon oatstraw

1 teaspoon lemon balm leaf

1 teaspoon black cohosh root

2 ounces vodka or apple cider vinegar

Put the herbs in a 2-ounce jar and add vodka or apple cider vinegar to fill. Close tightly and shake well. Keep in a pantry or cupboard for 3 weeks, shaking every day. Strain and transfer to a 2-ounce dropper bottle. Take 1 dropperful 3 times a day during week 3 of your cycle.

Hormones are often to blame when a new mother's emotions tip toward grief, melancholy, fear, and other challenging emotions. Living conditions, lack of emotional support, and inability to care for the infant can also play a role. I encourage any new mom to seek out support if she is feeling any of the above. There are state agencies, community groups, and support services out there to help. If none of those seem appealing, try your local herb shop, as they are often a source of information about free services that help with health and well-being. These recipes focus on balancing the emotions and promoting a positive state of mind.

## Postpartum Tea

2 ounces lemon balm

½ ounce nettle leaf

½ ounce motherwort leaf

½ ounce vitex leaf

½ ounce St. John's wort leaf and flower

Mix the herbs in a bowl and store in a glass jar. When needed, put 4 or 5 tablespoons in a quart jar and pour boiling water over the herbs to fill the jar. Let steep overnight and strain in the morning. Drink 3 cups a day.

## Postpartum Tincture

2 teaspoons St. John's wort
  leaf and flower

½ teaspoon vitex leaf

½ teaspoon lady's mantle leaf

½ teaspoon oatstraw

½ teaspoon schisandra berry

2 ounces vodka or apple cier vinegar

Put the herbs in a 2-ounce jar and add vodka or apple cider vinegar to fill. Close tightly and shake well. Keep in a pantry or cupboard for 3 weeks, shaking every day. Strain and transfer to a 2-ounce dropper bottle. Take 1 dropperful 3 times a day.

## Postpartum Capsules

½ ounce linden flower powder

½ ounce hawthorn berry powder

¼ ounce St. John's wort powder

¼ ounce skullcap leaf powder

¼ ounce rhodiola root powder

¼ ounce partridge berry powder

Mix the powdered herbs in a bowl and fill 200 empty capsules. Take 2 capsules 3 times a day.

## Uplift Essential Oil Blend

*Use this in your diffuser to infuse the air with uplifting scents to support you throughout the day.*

4 milliliters lavender essential oil

3 milliliters grapefruit essential oil

3 milliliters melissa essential oil

Blend the oils in a 10-milliliter bottle and add 5 drops to your diffuser when needed.

## ≡ PREGNANCY ≡

As joyous and exciting as pregnancy is, it often comes with a host of not-so-pleasant symptoms. These recipes are geared to help you keep the glow going and your eyes on the prize.

## Morning Sickness Lollipops

*Morning sickness can really make life a struggle, whether it occurs only at the beginning of the pregnancy or all throughout. Having a couple of go-to remedies can make a huge difference. If the flavors in this first recipe don't work for you, try different ones—maybe ginger or peppermint. You can also use this formula to make herbal ice cubes to suck on.*

3 tablespoons hibiscus flower

2 tablespoons orange peel

1 tablespoon licorice root

4 cups honey

Steep the herbs in 1 quart of hot water overnight. Strain in the morning and pour the liquid into a saucepan. Turn onto high and add the honey. Bring up the temperature to 300 degrees F and then quickly pour into a lollipop mold and put into the refrigerator. Don't forget the lollipop stick! Allow to fully cool and remove from the mold. Eat as desired.

## Anti-Nausea Tea

2 ounces calendula flower

1 ounce raspberry leaf

½ ounce red clover blossoms

¼ ounce ginger root

¼ ounce hop strobiles

Mix the herbs and store in a glass jar. Make tea by the cup. Steep 1 or 2 teaspoons in 10 ounces of hot water, covered, for 10 minutes. Drink to quickly quell the onset of nausea.

## Essential Oil Blend for Nausea

*Having this in a room or necklace diffuser can help to calm the nervous system and the nausea reflex.*

5 milliliters cardamom essential oil

2.5 milliliters spearmint essential oil

2.5 milliliters lemon essential oil

Blend the oils in a 10-milliliter essential oil bottle and add 5 drops to your diffuser as needed.

## Stretch Marks Oil

*Applying this topically can help to elasticize the skin and reduce the occurrence of stretch marks.*

2 tablespoons plantain leaf

2 tablespoons comfrey leaf

1 tablespoon lavender flower

1 tablespoon calendula flower

1 cup liquid coconut oil

20–40 drops sandalwood or

   helichrysum essential oil (optional)

Put the herbs in a glass baking dish and cover with coconut oil to a depth of 1 or 2 inches. Bake at 170 degrees F for 4 hours and then strain. You can add the essential oil if you'd like a scent and/or additional skin support. Apply 1 to 2 teaspoons twice daily where needed.

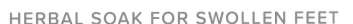

## HERBAL SOAK FOR SWOLLEN FEET

Get a foot basin from your local drugstore and fill it with warm water. Add 5 drops of cypress essential oil, 3 drops of lavender essential oil, and 10 drops of chamomile essential oil before soaking your feet.

## Anti-Swelling Tea

*Hydration is the best antidote to swelling of the hands, face, legs, ankles, and feet during pregnancy. Be sure your daily water intake is more than adequate. This herbal tea blend is for occasional support and relief, and can help mobilize the waterways and reduce swelling. It is not a cure for chronic edema while pregnant and shouldn't be used regularly.*

2 ounces dandelion leaf

1 ounce lemon balm leaf

½ ounce burdock root

½ ounce calendula flower

Mix the herbs in a bowl and store in a glass jar until needed. Make tea by the cup. Steep 1 or 2 teaspoons in 10 ounces of hot water, covered, for 10 minutes. Drink when needed for temporary relief.

## UTERINE FIBROIDS

Fibroids are a buildup of uterine tissue that can occur inside or outside the uterus. They can be provoked by xenoestrogens, menstrual irregularity, genetics, hormone imbalance, diet, stress, and environmental factors. They are not easy to treat and can range from not even being felt to causing pain and excessive bleeding or interfering with conceiving a child. They tend to shrink with pregnancy, which seems to indicate they are estrogen driven. Supporting your liver and endocrine system alongside the reproductive organs as well as diet and lifestyle treatments are necessary.

# CASTOR OIL FIBROID TREATMENT

Apply a castor oil pack to the abdomen twice daily to reduce inflammation and support the excretion of excess estrogen. Spread 2 tablespoons castor oil over the abdomen. Cover with a cotton towel and then a hot water bottle or heating pad. Relax for 30 to 45 minutes, or put on before bed and go to sleep.

## Fibroid-Shrinking Tea

2 ounces burdock root

½ ounce wild yam root

½ ounce yellow dock root

½ ounce licorice root

½ ounce angelica root

Mix the herbs in a bowl and store in a glass jar. When needed, put 4 or 5 tablespoons in a quart jar and pour boiling water over the herbs to fill the jar. Let steep overnight and strain in the morning. Drink 3 cups a day for 12 weeks and then reassess.

## Uterus-Support Tincture

*This tincture supports uterine tissue.*

2 teaspoons reishi mushroom

1 teaspoon turmeric root

1 teaspoon milk thistle

½ teaspoon plantain leaf

½ teaspoon yellow dock root

2 ounces vodka

Put the herbs in a 2-ounce jar and add vodka to fill. Close tightly and shake well. Keep in a pantry or cupboard for 3 weeks, shaking every day. Strain and transfer to a 2-ounce dropper bottle. Take 1 dropperful 3 times a day for 6 to 12 weeks.

# VAGINAL BACTERIAL INFECTIONS

The bacterial infection known as bacterial vaginosis (BV) can be a normal deviation of the flora of the vagina, but it's always best to be checked by a practitioner. Other vaginal infections can present with a stronger odor or symptoms that may require medical attention. Reconsider your diet and lifestyle if BV is a normal occurrence.

## Vaginal Wash for BV

1 ounce echinacea root

1 ounce chaparral leaf

1 ounce marshmallow root

1 ounce goldenseal root

Mix the herbs in a bowl and store in a glass jar. When needed, put 5 tablespoons in a quart jar and pour boiling water over the herbs to fill the jar. Let steep overnight and strain in the morning. Gently wash the vaginal area with the infusion twice daily for 5 to 7 days.

## BV-Quelling Tincture

2 teaspoons echinacea root

1 teaspoon skullcap leaf

1 teaspoon goldenseal root

½ teaspoon yarrow leaf and flower

½ teaspoon agrimony leaf

2 ounces vodka

Put the herbs in a 2-ounce jar and add vodka to fill. Close tightly and shake well. Keep in a pantry or cupboard for 3 weeks, shaking every day. Strain and transfer to a 2-ounce dropper bottle. Take 1 dropperful 3 times a day for 10 to 12 days.

## BV-Quelling Capsules

½ ounce pau d'arco leaf powder

½ ounce goldenseal root powder

¼ ounce black walnut hull powder

¼ ounce skullcap leaf powder

¼ ounce catnip leaf powder

¼ ounce lemon balm leaf powder

Mix the powdered herbs in a bowl and fill 200 empty capsules. Take 2 capsules twice a day until symptoms subside.

# ≡ VAGINAL INFECTIONS ≡

Vaginal infections occur when the pH of the vagina is thrown off by bacteria or candida. Women have healthy bacteria in the vagina that keeps the flora balanced, but when the balance is overthrown, symptoms arise such as odor, irritation, discharge, or pain. It's always best to see your health care provider if the symptoms are new to you, to rule out bacterial and sexually transmitted infections. Yeast infections are characterized by a white discharge that is thicker than normal and often accompanied by itchiness of the vaginal tissues.

## Yeast Infection Suppository

2 tablespoons powdered usnea

1 tablespoon yarrow powder

1 tablespoon goldenseal powder

1 tablespoon calendula powder

1 cup liquid coconut oil

40 drops tea tree essential oil

5 milliliters vitamin E oil

Put the herbs in a glass baking dish with the coconut oil and bake at 170 degrees F for 4 hours. Strain while warm and add the tea tree essential oil and the vitamin E oil. Pour into suppository molds and cool in the refrigerator to set. Pop out when hardened and keep in a glass jar in the refrigerator until needed. Insert one vaginally each night for 7 to 10 nights. Be sure to wear a pad at night to catch residual oil.

## Yeast-B-Gone Treatment

1 cup plain organic whole milk yogurt

1 teaspoon honey

20 drops melaleuca essential oil

10 drops lavender essential oil

As needed, mix the ingredients in a bowl and put into a glass jar for refrigerator storage. Apply 1 or 2 teaspoons to the vaginal opening and external tissues for relief of irritation and itch caused by a yeast infection.

## Yeast-Away Tea

1 ounce pau d'arco leaf

1 ounce chamomile flower

¾ ounce raspberry leaf

½ ounce yarrow leaf and flower

½ ounce goldenseal root

¼ ounce lavender flower

Mix the herbs in a bowl and store in a glass jar. When needed, put 4 or 5 tablespoons in a quart jar and pour boiling water over the herbs to fill the jar. Let steep overnight and strain in the morning. Drink 3 cups a day for 7 to 10 days.

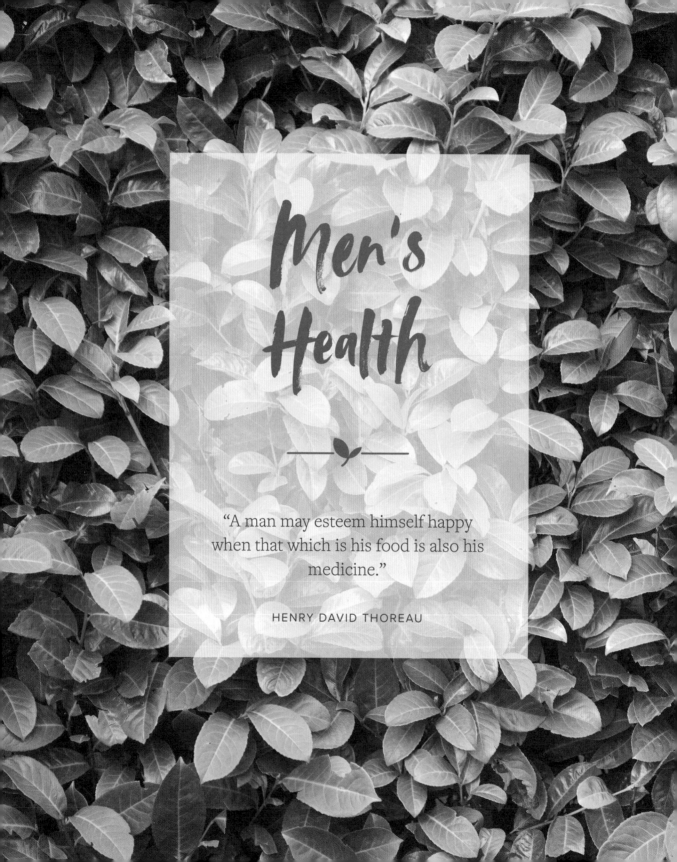

# Men's Health

"A man may esteem himself happy when that which is his food is also his medicine."

HENRY DAVID THOREAU

IT'S AN OLD STEREOTYPE that men never seek out help when sick or troubled about their health. Judging from my herb shop clientele, the message is getting through that we all need to care for ourselves in order to live long, healthy, and fulfilled lives. There are days at the shop when 90 percent of our customers are male and the staff are focused on their needs. I don't know why it happens that they all come on the same day, but I love these days. Working with men is particularly rewarding because they are often new to traditional medicine and we inevitably end up in the best conversations.

Certainly there are health concerns that are unique to men, but there are also those they share with women. Heart conditions top the charts for men, as they do for women,

## DIGESTION SUPPORT

Normal digestion checklist:

- occasional gas (FYI, the definition of occasional is infrequent or irregular)

- occasional bloating—perhaps once a week

- regular daily bowel movements (happening at approximately the same time each day, with stool that is formed, easy to pass, nongreasy/nonsticky, normal brown color)

- no stomach pain or abdominal cramping

- no being driven out of bed to have a bowel movement

If you experience deviations from any of the above, there is room for improvement. Review the recipes under "Indigestion" in the "Day-to-Day Health" section to help balance out your digestion and decrease digestive inflammation. Start with castor oil packs and digestive bitters to get the ball rolling toward better digestive function. Please see your health care provider if you are experiencing chronic pain, constipation, or loose stools.

but so do kidney and liver issues. Prostate health, gout, and low testosterone are common concerns, and men are also much more likely than women to experience depression. Though men and women may internalize and manifest stress differently, the underlying physiology is the same, and finding healthy outlets such as laughter, massage, music, and movement are just as important for men as for women. I encourage all men to read *The Male Herbal* by James Green, as it does an incredible job of helping men reconnect with the heritage of herbal medicine from which many have been disconnected.

## ═ GOUT ═

While gout does occur in women, it is predominantly a male issue. Gout is an inflammatory process caused by high levels of uric acid in the blood. The acid tends to settle in smaller joints of the body, and some medical professionals are now identifying it as a type of arthritis. It can cause sudden, severe episodes of pain, tenderness, redness, warmth, and swelling.

## Gout-Relief Tea

1 ounce white willow bark

1 ounce birch bark

½ ounce couch grass leaf

½ ounce gravel root

½ ounce juniper berry

½ ounce meadowsweet leaf

Mix the herbs in a bowl and store in a glass jar. When needed, put 4 or 5 tablespoons in a quart jar and pour boiling water over the herbs to fill the jar. Let steep overnight and strain in the morning. Drink 6 ounces every 3 hours for 3 days.

## Gout-Relief Tincture

*Have on hand for acute gout attacks.*

2 teaspoons birch bark

1 teaspoon nettle leaf

1 teaspoon devil's claw root

½ teaspoon pipsissewa leaf

½ teaspoon lobelia leaf

2 ounces vodka or applec cider vinegar

Put the herbs in a 2-ounce jar and add vodka or apple cider vinegar to fill. Close tightly and shake well. Keep in a pantry or cupboard for 3 weeks, shaking every day. Strain and transfer to a 2-ounce dropper bottle. Take 2 dropperfuls 4 times a day for 5 days.

## Salve for Gout

2 tablespoons birch bark

1 tablespoon club moss

1 tablespoon meadowsweet

1 tablespoon alder buckthorn bark

¾ cup olive oil

½ ounce beeswax

40 drops wintergreen essential oil

Put the herbs in a glass baking dish and cover with olive oil to a depth of 1 or 2 inches. Bake at 170 degrees F for 4 hours. Allow to cool and then strain. Pour the oil into a saucepan and add the beeswax. Gently heat until the beeswax is melted. Pour into container of your choice and add wintergreen essential oil. Apply to affected area as needed.

## ⮚ HEART HEALTH ⮘

"There is no fear in a shallow heart, because shallow hearts don't fall apart. But feeling hearts that truly care are fragile to the flow of air." I love this line from the song "The Fear in the Heart of a Man" by Tupac Shakur. Emotions and life patterns take a toll on the heart and I cannot deny the link between heart pathologies and emotional well-being I've seen repeatedly in my patients. I'm not saying heart disease doesn't occur without emotional imbalance, because, yes, genetics, diet, and lifestyle choices play a huge part, but so do emotions and in particular, self-worth. No matter who you are, what you've done in your life, I'm here to remind you that you are worthy of love, self-acceptance, joy, and so much more. Honor and nourish yourself daily. Stick up a quote on your refrigerator to remind yourself and use these herbal recipes as a meditation to remind yourself.

## Heart-Health Capsules

½ ounce hawthorn berry powder

½ ounce hawthorn leaf
 and flower powder

¼ ounce elderberry powder

¼ ounce grand cactus powder

¼ ounce horse chestnut powder

1 teaspoon lobelia leaf powder

Mix the powdered herbs in a bowl and fill 200 empty capsules. Take 2 capsules twice a day.

## Heart-Nourishing Syrup

2 cups hawthorn berry

1 cup black currant berry

¼ cup nutmeg

¼ cup cinnamon

4 cups water

1½ cups cane sugar or honey

¼ cup apple cider vinegar

Put all herbs in a saucepan with the water. Bring to a boil and reduce by half on a medium-low heat. Strain the herbs out and put the brew back into the pan. Add the sugar or honey and gently heat to mix if necessary, stirring continuously. Turn off the heat, add the apple cider vinegar, and allow to cool. Transfer to container of your choice and store in the refrigerator. Take 1 teaspoon daily.

## Strong Hearts Flower Essence

7 drops borage flower essence

7 drops holly flower essence

7 drops bleeding heart flower essence

7 drops aspen flower essence

distilled water

10 milliliters brandy

Blend the essences in a 1-ounce dropper bottle. Fill with distilled water and add the brandy for preservation. Take 4 drops 4 times a day.

# ≡ PROSTATE HEALTH ≡

Does it seem inevitable that every man will experience prostate issues as he ages? Our Western medical practitioners say yes, it is a natural part of the aging process, but I say no. Just as for any body part, taking a proactive approach to the prostate will result in healthy functioning. The prostate is just as susceptible to toxins in our environment and food as a woman's reproductive system is. Men have just as much need for exercise to liberate stored hormones as women do. A proper balance of hormones and the elimination of by-products and waste is necessary.

While little research is available, one can only guess that from a hormonal perspective, men go through an experience similar to women's menopause as they age. As potency declines, hormone levels must shift, and as hormones decrease, hormone receptors in the male reproductive system also decrease. When the prostate and its surrounding muscles are no longer being flexed as they once were, just as with anything, they will become lax and/or stagnant. Ancient Chinese medical philosophy recommends that men continue to ejaculate at least once a week after age fifty-five.

## Prostate-Tonic Capsules

1 ounce red root powder

1 ounce nettle root powder

½ ounce white pond lily powder

½ ounce dandelion root powder

½ ounce dandelion leaf powder

½ ounce gentian powder

Mix the powdered herbs in a bowl and fill 200 empty capsules. Take 2 capsules twice a day.

## Prostate-Pain Tincture

2 teaspoons sumac berry

1 teaspoon turmeric root

1 teaspoon chickweed leaf

½ teaspoon saw palmetto berry

½ teaspoon nettle leaf

2 ounces vodka

Put the herbs in a 2-ounce jar and add vodka to fill. Close tightly and shake well. Keep in a pantry or cupboard for 3 weeks, shaking every day. Strain and transfer to a 2-ounce dropper bottle. Take 1 to 2 dropperfuls as needed. If pain increases or remains after 1 week, please consult your primary health care practitioner.

## Prostate Massage Oil

2 tablespoons hawthorn leaf and flower

1 tablespoon barberry

1 tablespoon calendula flower

¾ cup pumpkin seed

15 drops fennel seed essential oil

5 drops peppermint essential oil

2 cups olive oil

Put the herbs in a glass baking dish and cover the herbs with oil to depth of 1 or 2 inches. Bake at 170 degrees F for 4 hours. Allow to cool and then strain. Add essential oils and transfer into a squeeze bottle with a dispenser cap. Use 1 to 2 teaspoons to massage the perineum area several times a week.

# ⟹ STAMINA AND IMPOTENCE ⟸

Sometimes it's all in the self-motivation to get the sexual stimulus going, while other times the body doesn't seem to want to cooperate. Herbs to boost libido and improve erectile function and stamina have been used for centuries.

## Go-Time Tincture

2 teaspoons yohimbe bark

1 teaspoon epimedium leaf

½ teaspoon passionflower leaf

½ teaspoon hops strobiles

½ teaspoon ginkgo leaf

½ teaspoon gotu kola leaf

2 ounces vodka

Put the herbs in a 2-ounce jar and add vodka to fill. Close tightly and shake well. Keep in a pantry or cupboard for 3 weeks, shaking every day. Strain and transfer to a 2-ounce dropper bottle. Take 1 or 2 dropperfuls 30 minutes before desired sexual activity and again right before.

## Libido-Tonic Capsules

½ ounce maca root powder

½ ounce tribulus leaf powder

¼ ounce epimedium leaf powder

¼ ounce raspberry leaf powder

¼ ounce nettle leaf powder

¼ ounce spirulina powder

Mix the powdered herbs in a bowl and fill 200 empty capsules. Take 2 capsules twice a day.

## ═ URINATION FREQUENCY ═

When the prostate is enlarged, there are often uncomfortable urination symptoms. This can include difficulty initiating urination, pain with urination, frequency, or incomplete urination with a dribbling effect. Herbs can help reducing the swelling and inflammation so you can be more comfortable.

## Rooting-for-Your-Bladder Tea

1 ounce burdock root

1 ounce fenugreek seed

1 ounce yucca root

¼ ounce sassafras root bark

¼ ounce sarsaparilla root

¼ ounce saw palmetto berry

¼ ounce licorice root

Mix the herbs in a bowl and store in a glass jar. When needed, put 4 to 5 tablespoons in a quart jar and pour boiling water over the herbs to fill the jar. Let steep overnight and strain in the morning. Drink 3 cups a day, hot or cold, sweetened with honey if desired.

## Bladder-Tone Tincture

2 teaspoons goldenrod leaf

1 teaspoon devil's claw root

½ teaspoon raspberry leaf

½ teaspoon comfrey leaf

½ teaspoon gotu kola leaf

½ teaspoon safflower flower

2 ounces vodka or apple cider vinegar

Put the herbs in a 2-ounce jar and add vodka or apple cider vinegar to fill. Close tightly and shake well. Keep in a pantry or cupboard for 3 weeks, shaking every day. Strain and transfer to a 2-ounce dropper bottle. Take 1 dropperful 3 times a day.

# Care for Babies and Children

—🌿—

"Why try to explain miracles to your
kids when you can just have them
plant a garden?"

ROBERT BRAULT

I GREW UP IN THE ANTIBIOTIC ERA and as a child probably took three or four courses of antibiotics each winter. Whenever my throat hurt, my ears ached, or my fever shot up, I would be given the same amoxicillin. Sometimes it was warranted, but many times it was not. As I grew older and began studying herbs and nature cure traditions, I became more comfortable identifying when I was able to treat myself and when I did indeed need to see my health care practitioner. By the time I had my first child, using herbs seemed only natural to me.

Children respond so much more quickly than adults to medicines of any type. Just a little yarrow and peppermint tea brought my daughter's fevers down, and a little cleavers oil to the throat diminished swollen glands. When I caught a nasty cold when my son was

## GUIDELINES FOR TREATING CHILDREN AND BABIES

- If cold symptoms are present, get on it. Don't delay in treating.

- Always treat a cough aggressively.

- Take a look at what you're wearing before you go outside with your baby or child. If you are wearing a heavy coat and winter hat, your child should be too. Yes, kids run warm, but leaving them exposed to wind and cold is inviting a cold to come in.

- Don't overdress for bedtime.

- Use essential oils in a diffuser to prevent the domino effect when one member of the family gets sick.

- When one member of the family gets sick, be proactive with immune-boosting herbs for everyone else.

just four weeks old, I drank a tea of boneset, elderflower, echinacea root, and peppermint to fight it and provide my son the protective benefits through my breast milk. I have found that most children relate to plants as healing medicine and often want to know what the herb looks like and how it works. Having this cooperative relationship with patients who want to actively participate in their healing process is quite rewarding.

Many customers come to my herb shop for the first time when they become parents. They are seeking gentle but effective ways to help their children move through day-to-day issues and to relieve discomfort. Herbs can offer a supportive approach to many families' daily health needs. Encourage your children to share the experience with you as you make the recipes in this section. Even when they are babies, you can show them the herbs and how to take them. Our kids are always watching us and gain from positive demonstration.

## ≡ BAD DREAMS AND SCARY THINGS ≡

Whether a movie or a bad uncle has put scary thoughts into your child's mind, helping them through the very real fear is necessary. Never brush off a child's fear as insignificant. Always do your best to have patience as you support them through to safety.

## Monster-Rid Sachet

Fill a sachet with protective herbs of various traditions such as bearberry and cat's claw and give it to the child to denote the protection they will receive from having the herbs close to them. Sprinkle a pinch of herbs on all four corners of the bed and announce that no monster shall be allowed to pass there.

## No-Monsters-Allowed Spray

Fill a 2-ounce spray bottle with distilled water and add essential oils of your choice. I suggest using relaxing oils verses stimulating ones. Spray the spray each night at bedtime, ensuring you get under the bed and in the closet.

Learning to hold your bladder through the night after years of relaxing it at free will can be hard! Some children struggle with the reflex, and the key to success is compassion. As frustrating or inconvenient as it may be, offering support and a hug to children when they are learning this transition is so important. Bedwetting is often involuntary. Sometimes using herbs to tone the bladder and the pelvic bowl is all that is needed.

## Bladder-Tone Drops

2 teaspoons plantain leaf

1 teaspoon raspberry leaf

1 teaspoon cornsilk

½ teaspoon burdock root

½ teaspoon catnip leaf

2 ounces vegetable glycerin

Put the herbs in a 2-ounce jar and add vegetable glycerin to fill. Close tightly and shake well. Keep in a pantry or cupboard for 3 weeks, shaking every day. Strain and transfer to a 2-ounce dropper bottle. Give 2 dropperfuls at bedtime.

## Bladder-Tone Oil

*When my daughter was first trying to sleep without diapers and training pants at bedtime, we did a little ritual each night. After book time we'd rub a little oil onto her belly and talk to her bladder, saying things like "Hello bladder! I'd like to try to hold my pee all night tonight. It's okay if you get too full and can't, because we can always try again tomorrow. Just know I believe you can do it and someday you will." Then I'd tuck her in for the night.*

2 tablespoons plantain leaf

1 tablespoon comfrey leaf

1 tablespoon chamomile flower

1 tablespoon rose petals

¾ cup olive oil

lavender essential oil

Put the herbs in a glass baking dish and cover with olive oil to a depth of 1 or 2 inches. Bake at 170 degrees F for 4 hours. Allow to cool and then strain. Pour into container of your choice and add a few drops of lavender essential oil. Rub 1 teaspoon over the abdomen at night before bed.

# DOSAGE GUIDELINES FOR CHILDREN

Any parent who is just learning about herbs needs some guidance to determine the appropriate quantities of herbs for children. The goal is to use a safe quantity of herbs but also use enough to be effective. Use these dosage tables to determine the appropriate quantity of herbs to give a child. And use the dosages given for each of the specific recipes in this section, even if they don't exactly match these general guidelines.

## TEA DOSAGES FOR CHILDREN

(if adult dosage is 1 cup, or 8 ounces)

| | |
|---|---|
| Younger than 1 year | ½ to 3 teaspoons |
| 2 to 4 years | 1 to 4 ounces |
| 4 to 7 years | 2 to 4 ounces |
| 7 to 11 years | 4 to 6 ounces |

## TINCTURE DOSAGES FOR CHILDREN

(if adult dosage is 2 dropperfuls, or 60 drops)

| | |
|---|---|
| Younger than 3 months* | 2 drops |
| 3 to 6 months* | 3 drops |
| 6 to 9 months* | 4 drops |
| 9 to 12 months* | 5 drops |
| 12 to 18 months* | 7 drops |
| 18 to 24 months* | 8 drops |
| 2 to 3 years* | 10 drops |
| 3 to 4 years | 12 drops |
| 4 to 6 years | 15 drops |
| 6 to 9 years | 24 drops |
| 9 to 12 years | 30 drops (1 dropperful) |

*GLYCERINE-ONLY TINCTURES FOR 2 YEARS AND YOUNGER

## CHILD DOSAGES

age 12 or older

| Preparation | Dosage |
|---|---|
| Glycerin tinctures | 1 dropperful, 3 or 4 times per day |
| Syrups | 1 teaspoon, 3 to 6 times per day, depending on case |

You can also use two equations to determine dosage of any herbal medicine to achieve the percentage of the adult dosage appropriate for a child:

❧ YOUNG'S RULE Add 12 to the child's age, and divide the child's age by this total. For example, to determine the dosage for a 4-year-old: 4 + 12 = 16. Then 4 ÷ 16 = 0.25, or one-fourth of the adult dosage.

❧ COWLING'S RULE Divide the child's age at his or her next birthday by 24. For example, the dosage for a child who is 3, turning 4 at his next birthday, would be 4 ÷ 24 = 0.16, or about one-sixth of the adult dosage.

# ⩵ CHICKEN POX ⩵

If your children should fall ill with chicken pox (vaccinated or not), making them comfortable is the most difficult task. We've all seen kids with oven mitts taped onto their hands to prevent scarring from scratching. Try these recipes to help topically and from the inside out.

## Oatmeal Herbal Bath

2 cups oatmeal (use gluten free if needed)

1 cup baking soda

1 cup chamomile flower

½ cup basil leaf

½ cup mullein leaf

Get a large muslin bag and fill it with the ingredients. Run a warm, not hot, bath. Allow the muslin bag to soak in the water as the faucet is running. Be sure to fill up the tub enough so the children can fully submerge themselves. Allow soaking in the bath for 20 minutes.

## Pox Spot Treatment

1 ounce plantain leaf powder

1 ounce chickweed leaf powder

½ ounce spilanthes flower powder

¼ ounce mullein leaf powder

¼ ounce goldenseal root powder

Mix the powders in a bowl and store in a glass jar. Put 1 tablespoon of the powdered blend in a bowl and add enough hot water to make a thick paste. Dip a Q-tip into the paste and dab onto each pox sore for temporary relief.

## Virus-Fighting Drops

2 teaspoons reishi mushroom

1 teaspoon elderberry

1 teaspoon lemon balm leaf

½ teaspoon spilanthes flower

½ teaspoon yarrow flower

1½ ounces vegetable glycerin

½ ounce apple cider vinegar

Put the herbs in a 2-ounce jar and add the vegetable glycerin and apple cider vinegar to fill. Close tightly and shake well. Keep in a pantry or cupboard for 3 weeks, shaking every day. Strain and transfer to a 2-ounce dropper bottle. Give 10 to 30 drops every few hours.

# ⇛ COLIC ⇚

Colic is one of the rites of passage for parenthood. If you've ever experienced this with your child, you know what I mean. Gas, bloating, constipation—all of it is incredibly difficult for a baby and doing the best you can to support them until their digestive system matures takes great strength. You can offer herbal support with the following recipes. I would also recommend speaking to your health care provider regarding the use of l-glutamine and probiotics, as I've seen them provide valuable support.

## Tummy Rub

½ ounce lavender flower

¼ ounce fennel seed

1 cup castor oil

Put the herbs in a glass baking dish and cover with castor oil to a depth of 1 or 2 inches. Bake at 170 degrees F for 4 hours. Allow to cool and then strain and transfer to container of your choice. Rub 1 or 2 teaspoons over the entire abdomen 3 times a day. I would typically apply a little at each diaper change.

## Colic-Calm Tea

*By the time my son was 8 months, he'd open his mouth like a little bird to receive this tea via dropper.*

2 ½ ounces chamomile flower

1 ounce catnip leaf

½ ounce fennel seed

Mix the herbs in a bowl and store in a glass jar. Make tea by the cup. Steep 1 or 2 teaspoons in 10 ounces of hot water, covered, for 10 minutes. Give 1 to 2 dropperfuls several times a day.

# ≡ CONSTIPATION ≡

New food, not enough water, food allergies, and imbalanced digestive function can all lead to constipation. Start with more water and then move to one of these remedies. They say each child is different, and my daughter and son have definitely proved that. My daughter pooped three to six times a day as a baby, whereas my son often went days on end with no bowel movement. My son didn't display any signs of discomfort or distress—only I did. As any naturopath can tell you, pooping is a major part of health, but some babies' digestive systems take longer to develop. When children get a bit older and are going to the bathroom on their own, it is important to monitor them at times to ensure bowel movements are happening and are within normal boundaries of timing, color, and consistency, and are without pain.

## Conk-Out-Constipation Candy

*These are great to have on hand and are a fun and tasty way to convince a child to take herbs.*

1½ ounces triphala powder

½ ounce flax seed powder

¼ ounce marshmallow powder

¼ ounce fennel powder

⅛ ounce licorice powder

1–2 cups nut butter of choice

¼ cup honey

Mix the powders together and add the nut butter and then the honey. You can also add a little cinnamon, vanilla, or carob if you'd like. Roll into 1-inch balls and keep in the refrigerator. Give 1 or 2 candies as needed.

## Move-It-Gently Tea

2 ounces catnip leaf

1 ounce chamomile flower

½ ounce fennel seed

¼ ounce buckthorn

¼ ounce licorice root

Mix the herbs in a bowl and store in a glass jar. Make tea by the cup. Steep 1 or 2 teaspoons in 10 ounces of hot water, covered, for 10 minutes. Give 1 cup as needed.

# CASTOR OIL CONSTIPATION TREATMENT

My go-to remedy for constipation in children is a castor oil pack on the abdomen. It seems to always do the trick. I often put one on my son's belly before bed and sure enough, after breakfast in the morning he finds relief. Spread 2 tablespoons castor oil over the abdomen. Cover with a cotton towel and then a hot water bottle or heating pad. Leave on all night.

## COUGHS

I'm sure I've said it a hundred times: always always always treat a cough at the first sign of it. This is immensely easier than trying to rid the body of it after it has taken hold. Treat the cough itself with appropriate herbs to alleviate the spasm, irritation, and/or phlegm while simultaneously treating the immune and respiratory systems.

### Herbal Cough Syrup

1 ounce coltsfoot leaf

½ ounce mullein leaf

½ ounce pleurisy root

½ ounce wild cherry bark

½ ounce horehound leaf

½ ounce marshmallow root

½ ounce goldenseal root

8 cups water

3 cups cane sugar or honey

¼ cup apple cider vinegar

Put the herbs in a saucepan with the water, bring to a boil, and reduce by half on a medium-low heat. Strain the herbs out and put the brew back into the pan. Add the sugar or honey and gently heat to mix if necessary, stirring continuously. Turn off the heat, add the apple cider vinegar, and allow to cool. Transfer to container of your choice. Give 1 to 2 teaspoons 3 times a day.

## Cough-Killer Tea

1 ounce hyssop leaf

1 ounce peppermint leaf

½ ounce coltsfoot leaf

½ ounce mullein leaf

½ ounce marshmallow root

½ ounce licorice root

Mix the herbs in a bowl and store in a glass jar. Make tea by the cup. Steep 1 or 2 teaspoons in 10 ounces of hot water, covered, for 10 minutes. Give 2 or 3 cups a day. If the patient is a baby who is being breastfed, the mother can drink the tea to help support the baby. After 6 months of age you can give 1-teaspoon doses if desired.

## Respiratory-Support Tincture

2 teaspoons elecampane root

1 teaspoon goldenseal root

½ teaspoon echinacea root

½ teaspoon rosemary leaf

2 ounces vegetable glycerin

Put the herbs in a 2-ounce jar and add vegetable glycerin to fill. Close tightly and shake well. Keep in a pantry or cupboard for 3 weeks, shaking every day. Strain and transfer to a 2-ounce dropper bottle. Give 1 dropperful 3 times a day at the first sign of a cough or respiratory infection.

# ≡ CRADLE CAP ≡

Cradle cap is the common, and benign, condition of baby dandruff. It is often yellow due to the oily secretions on the head, and it can have a waxy appearance. If cradle cap is the diagnosis, it typically passes on its own, but it can be distressing for some parents. I've rarely seen it bother a child. Try your best not to pick at it as that can lead to irritation and sometimes infection if you've got bacteria under your fingernails.

## Cradle-Cap Wash

*Use this blend to gently wash your baby's head to free loose pieces.*

1 ounce dandelion root

1 ounce fenugreek seed

½ ounce red clover blossom

½ ounce comfrey leaf

Mix the herbs in a bowl and store in a glass jar. When needed, put 5 tablespoons in a quart jar and pour boiling water over the herbs to fill the jar. Let steep 1 hour and then strain. You can keep the herbs to reuse. Soak a small cotton cloth in the infusion and wrap it around the baby's head. Then while the baby is in the bath, gently pour the infusion over the head, ensuring you've warmed it up so that it is comfortable.

## Cradle-Cap Oil

*Applying this gentle oil to the head can help reduce flakes and noticeable irritation.*

2 teaspoons chamomile flower

1 teaspoon lavender flower

1 teaspoon burdock root

1 teaspoon red clover blossom

¾ cup grapeseed oil

30 drops sandalwood essential oil

Put the herbs in a glass baking dish and cover with olive oil to a depth of 1 or 2 inches. Bake at 170 degrees F for 4 hours. Allow to cool and then strain. Pour into container of choice and add essential oil. Apply to the head as needed.

# ≡ CROUP ≡

Croup is a respiratory infection that often begins as an ordinary cold but then sinks into the lungs. It is characterized by the sound of a hard or barklike cough. Typically it is also worse at night. It is viral, so try also the Virus-Fighting Drops under "Chicken Pox."

## Croup-Quell Drops

2 teaspoons hyssop leaf

½ ounce mullein leaf

½ ounce elderflower

½ ounce elecampane root

½ ounce elderberry

1½ ounces vegetable glycerin

½ ounce apple cider vinegar

Put the herbs in a 2-ounce jar and add vegetable glycerin and apple cider vinegar to fill. Close tightly and shake well. Keep in a pantry or cupboard for 3 weeks, shaking every day. Strain and transfer to a 2-ounce dropper bottle. Give 10 to 30 drops every few hours.

## Croup-B-Gone Vapor Balm

*This aromatic balm is a great to fight the viral load and open up the lungs.*

2 tablespoons marjoram leaf

1 tablespoon lemon peel

1 tablespoon rosemary leaf

1 tablespoon lavender flower

¾ cup olive oil

½ ounce beeswax

40 drops rosemary essential oil

Put the herbs in a glass baking dish and cover with olive oil to a depth of 1 or 2 inches. Bake at 170 degrees F for 4 hours. Allow to cool and then strain. Pour the oil into a saucepan and add the beeswax. Gently heat until the beeswax is melted. Pour into container of your choice and add the essential oil. Rub on the chest and feet before bed.

# ≡ CUTS AND SCRAPES ≡

Teaching your little ones to care for themselves whenever they get a cut or scape is a great start to future self-care. Add an essential oil to scent the salve that they pick out. Better yet, make the salve together and let them create their own label. Most of the following herbs are antibacterial and antimicrobial to fight off infection and promote healing of the skin.

## Cuts and Scrapes Salve

2 tablespoons calendula flower

1 tablespoon elderflower

1 tablespoon comfrey leaf

1 tablespoon lavender flower

1 cup olive oil

Put the herbs in a glass baking dish and cover with olive oil to a depth of 1 or 2 inches. Bake at 170 degrees F for 4 hours. Allow to cool and then strain. Rub into cuts and scrapes as needed.

## Boo-Boo Spray

*Spray this on a cut or scape when your child won't let you get near with a washcloth to wash the wound.*

1 tablespoon calendula flower

1½ ounces witch hazel extract

½ ounce aloe vera gel

50 drops lavender essential oil

Steep the calendula flowers in 6 ounces hot water for 1 hour. Strain and add 2 ounces of the water to a 4-ounce spray bottle. Add the witch hazel, aloe vera, and essential oil. Shake well and spray on skin as needed.

Diaper rash is a common occurrence in babies and if not treated can be very uncomfortable for your little one. The goal is to heal the tissue and create a barrier to further irritation. This is why so many commercial brands use petroleum, as it is an excellent waterproof barrier. Unfortunately, its use comes with a host of concerns. Luckily there are many natural options.

## Baby Bum Powder

½ ounce arrowroot powder

¼ ounce kaolin clay

¼ ounce lavender flower powder

¼ ounce comfrey leaf powder

¼ ounce marshmallow root powder

Mix the powders in a bowl and put into a spice shaker jar. Lightly dust the diaper area, getting the powder into the folds of skin. If a rash is present that is looking irritated, add ¼ ounce goldenseal root powder to the formula.

## D-Rash Herbal Ointment

½ ounce comfrey leaf

¼ ounce calendula flower

¼ ounce chickweed leaf

1 cup castor oil

1–2 ounces lanolin

2 teaspoons beeswax

2 ounces aloe vera gel

Put the herbs in a glass baking dish and cover with castor oil to a depth of 1 or 2 inches. Bake at 170 degrees F for 4 hours. Strain and pour the oil into a saucepan. Add the lanolin and beeswax and heat on low if needed to melt. Stir slowly until blended. Turn off the heat and add the aloe vera gel. Transfer to a squeeze bottle and apply with each diaper change when rash is present.

# ≈ DIARRHEA ≈

Diarrhea in children is often a sign that something is off. It may be an indication that your little one is about to come down with a bug, as viruses are a common cause of diarrhea, it can be a part of teething, or it could just be something they ate. Either way, the diarrhea process is the body's way of shedding whatever is occurring in its best attempt to move on with life. Chronic diarrhea must be investigated, as dehydration and nutrient deficiencies can come quickly in little ones.

## Anti-Diarrhea Drops

2 teaspoons Oregon grape root

1 teaspoon calendula flower

½ teaspoon slippery elm bark

½ teaspoon goldenseal root

2 ounces vegetable glycerin

Put the herbs in a 2-ounce jar and add vegetable glycerin to fill. Close tightly and shake well. Keep in a pantry or cupboard for 3 weeks, shaking every day. Strain and transfer to a 2-ounce dropper bottle. Give 1 to 2 dropperfuls 3 times a day.

## Diarrhea-Stop Tea

2 ounces raspberry leaf

½ ounce calendula flower

½ ounce Oregon grape root

¼ ounce marshmallow root

¼ ounce sage leaf

¼ ounce cinnamon chips

¼ ounce licorice root

Mix the herbs in a bowl and store in a glass jar. Make tea by the cup. Steep 1 or 2 teaspoons in 10 ounces of hot water, covered, for 10 minutes. Give 3 cups a day as needed.

## Belly-Calming Oil

2 teaspoons cramp bark

2 teaspoons hop strobiles

1 teaspoon ginger root

¾ cup castor oil

40 drops fennel essential oil

Put the herbs in a glass baking dish and pour castor oil over the herbs to a depth of 1 or 2 inches. Bake at 170 degrees F for 4 hours. Allow to cool and then strain. Transfer to bottle of your choice and add the essential oil. Apply 1 to 2 teaspoons of the oil to the belly. Cover with a cotton towel and then a hot water bottle or heating pad.

## ≡ EARACHES ≡

See "Earaches" in the "Immune Defense" section.

## ≡ EYE DISCHARGE ≡

When babies' eyes are goopy, rinsing with breast milk can be helpful. Squeezing a little out into a cup and gently pouring it into the eye can help you avoid the situation described by my patients where she tries to squirt it above the eye so it can gently roll down into her baby's eye but she squirts it full-on into the eye, causing a sudden surprise and a scream. You can also try the following recipe.

## Gentle Eye Rinse

2 ounces chamomile flower

1 ounce calendula flower

½ ounce chickweed leaf

½ ounce anise seed

Mix the herbs in a bowl and store in a glass jar. When needed, put 4 tablespoons in a pint jar and pour boiling water over the herbs to fill the jar. Let steep 1 hour and then strain. Apply using a cotton pad or ball, 3 times a day.

# ═ FEVER ═

A true fever in a child can be a very scary experience. Even as a doctor, I have had moments of deep concern when my children have spiked high fevers. When my daughter experienced her first multiple-day fever of 105 F, I questioned myself repeatedly despite my training. I called her pediatrician, who again reminded me that what I was describing was a normal bug. Yes, kids' fevers tend to go high and that is almost always normal, but when you see your child suffering like this it can be a hopeless feeling, and fears can quickly take over. If you decide to reach for the kids' ibuprofen even though you believe in living as naturally as possible, please don't view that as a failure. It isn't going to derail your values should you decide to use modern medicine at certain times as well as the remedies described here.

## Fever-Reliever Tea

*This tea helps to gently reduce fever and provide comfort to the patient.*

1 ¾ ounces yarrow leaf and flower

1 ounce peppermint leaf

½ ounce echinacea root

½ ounce boneset leaf

¼ ounce licorice root

Mix the herbs in a bowl and store in a glass jar. Make tea by the cup. Steep 1 or 2 teaspoons in 10 ounces of hot water, covered, for 10 minutes. You may want to start by offering just 6 ounces of the tea. Getting kids to drink tea when they aren't feeling well may take some encouraging, but once they make the connection to how it makes them feel better, it'll get easier.

## Cooling Fomentation

40 drops peppermint essential oil

Add the essential oil to cool water in a basin and soak a cotton cloth in it. Wring it out and apply to the forehead.

## Fever-Reliever Diffuser Blend

3 milliliters basil essential oil

1 milliliter peppermint essential oil

1 milliliter eucalyptus essential oil

Blend the oils in a 5-milliliter bottle and add 5 drops to your room diffuser.

## ≡ FUSSINESS ≡

Fussiness can happen at any age. Sometimes babies and kids are physically uncomfortable, but many times it is due to overfatigue, overhunger, or overstimulation. These recipes can help bring a moment of calm so you can assess and move forward again in the direction needed.

## Child-Calming Massage Oil

½ ounce lavender flower

¼ ounce rose petals

¼ ounce chamomile flower

¾–1 cup olive oil

40 drops lavender essential oil

Put the herbs in a glass baking dish and cover with olive oil to a depth of 1 or 2 inches. Bake at 170 degrees F for 4 hours. Allow to cool and then strain. Pour into container of your choice and add essential oil. Rub all over the body after a bath, or just a little on the temples anytime.

## Child-Calming Syrup

2 ounces hawthorn berry

1 ounce rose petals

1 ounce chamomile flower

8 cups water

3 cups cane sugar or honey

¼ cup apple cider vinegar

Put the herbs in a saucepan with the water. Bring to a boil and reduce by half on a medium-low heat. Strain herbs out and put the brew back into the pan. Add sugar or honey and gently heat to mix if necessary, stirring continuously. Turn off the heat, add the apple cider vinegar, and allow to cool. Then transfer to container of your choice and store in the refrigerator. Give 1 teaspoon as desired or 30 minutes before bedtime.

## Calming Bedtime Sachet

*This one I do with other children, allowing them to pick the scents they'd prefer to have.*

lavender flower

lemon balm leaf

catnip leaf

fennel seed

cinnamon stick

rose petals

chamomile flower

scraps of fabric cut into 2-inch-
   by-4-inch pieces

Double the fabric over and sew it inside out on three sides and then turn it right side out. Fill the pocket with herbs of your choice, ensuring not to overfill. Sew it closed and place it under the pillow at bedtime.

## ═ HEAD COLDS ═

When your little one can't breathe, no one is sleeping at night. My son recently had a cold with so much phlegm in his little nose that he'd wake up with both nose holes sealed over. Getting the mucus to thin out and drain helps to clear the head, and using essential oils to stimulate the olfactory can move that cold out of the body.

## Decongestion Tea

1 ounce peppermint leaf

1 ounce spearmint leaf

1 ounce elderflower

½ ounce echinacea root

½ ounce ginger root

Mix the herbs in a bowl and store in a glass jar. Make tea by the cup. Steep 1 or 2 teaspoons in 10 ounces of hot water, covered, for 10 minutes. Have the child drink while warm.

## Cold-Breakup Tincture

2 teaspoons elderberry

1 teaspoon horehound leaf

1 teaspoon boneset leaf

½ teaspoon goldenseal root

½ teaspoon peppermint leaf

2 ounces vegetable glycerin

Put the herbs in a 2-ounce jar and add vegetable glycerin to fill. Close tightly and shake well. Keep in a pantry or cupboard for 3 weeks, shaking every day. Strain and transfer to a 2-ounce dropper bottle. Give 1-2 dropperfuls 4 times a day.

## Decongestant Chest Rub

2 tablespoons eucalyptus leaf

1 tablespoon rosemary leaf

1 tablespoon mullein leaf

¾ cup olive oil

½ ounce beeswax

40 drops white thyme essential oil

20 drops pine essential oil

Put the herbs in a glass baking dish and cover with olive oil to a depth of 1 or 2 inches. Bake at 170 degrees F for 4 hours. Allow to cool and then strain. Pour the oil into a saucepan and add the beeswax. Gently heat until the beeswax is melted. Pour into container of your choice and add the essential oils. Rub on the chest as needed.

## GINGER TEA BATH WITH ROSEMARY ESSENTIAL OIL

Never underestimate the power of a bath. Gently simmering a few slices of fresh ginger root in water for tea to drink while in a bath with 2 to 3 drops of rosemary essential oil can really open up the nasal passageways.

# THE FACTS OF LICE

- An examination of the hair is completely ineffective unless you have more lice than I'm comfortable thinking about. Instead, apply some coconut oil to the scalp and then use a lice comb to scrape in one stroke along the top of head.

- Many kids (and adults) don't have excessive itching with lice, which makes regular checks necessary while children are in their younger years.

- Lice can only be transferred by head-to-head contact. They cannot jump or survive off of the head. They don't migrate to beards.

- Lice can hold their breath for something like 16 hours. So much for using coconut oil to try to suffocate them.

- Commercial and prescription products are now ineffective as the lice have adapted. Great.

- The key isn't what you put on your hair but using a special lice comb. When I received my lice removal treatment, my scalp was tender for 2 days from the scraping close to the scalp to ensure removal of all lice and nits. Oh—and nits are often brown, not white. The white nits are after they have hatched.

- You don't need to wash everything like a crazy person. When I found the first louse on my daughter's head, I literally began piling up every washable item we'd touched in the last week. But what I learned is to wash bedding, coats, and clothes recently worn but simply throw most things in the dryer as the heat kills the lice.

- It is normal for your head to still itch 1 to 2 days after the treatment as the histamine reaction from the lice bites is still resounding.

- Recheck 3 days after treatment to ensure you've eradicated the lice.

# ≡ HEAD LICE ≡

When my daughter and I fell victim to head lice, I'll admit I was freaked out. I went to the professionals to learn everything I could. What most parents don't know is that lice have adapted to over-the-counter commercial treatments, meaning herbal remedies may actually be more effective in many cases.

## Lice-Killer Oil

3 ounces olive oil

3 ounces neem oil

2 ounces coconut oil

40 drops peppermint essential oil

20 drops eucalyptus essential oil

20 drops rosemary essential oil

20 drops lavender essential oil

Mix the ingredients together and put into an 8-ounce squeeze bottle with applicator tip. First brush the hair free of all tangles. Squirt a moderate amount on the head in sections and begin the combing process. You need to do the combing in sections and scrape the lice comb along the scalp. After each pass, clean the comb using a paper towel. Don't look if you get queasy with bugs. Go slowly and be super-dooper thorough. Once you've repeatedly done a thorough scraping of the scalp, you can wash your hair.

# ≡ IMPETIGO ≡

Scratching and picking is almost inevitable with kiddos. When they continue to scratch a scab, it becomes vulnerable to bacteria from under their fingernails or the environment they are playing in. When you see a scab with a honey-crusted appearance, you may be dealing with impetigo, a bacterial skin infection that leads to red sores that can break open, ooze fluid, and develop a yellow-brown crust. It most often is caused by the Staphylococcus aureus bacteria and is rarely serious unless it goes unnoticed for prolonged periods of time. Using antibacterial herbs topically as well as internally usually resolves the situation.

# Antibacterial Salve

2 tablespoons calendula flower

1 tablespoon comfrey leaf

½ tablespoon myrrh resin

½ tablespoon goldenseal root

¾ cup olive oil

½ ounce beeswax

60 drops lavender essential oil

Put the herbs in a glass baking dish and cover with olive oil to a depth of 1 or 2 inches. Bake at 170 degrees F for 4 hours. Allow to cool and then strain. Pour the oil into a saucepan and add the beeswax. Gently heat until the beeswax is melted. Pour into container of your choice and add the essential oil. Apply to the skin as needed.

# Bacteria-Stop Tea

2 ounces peppermint leaf

1 ounce calendula flower

½ ounce yarrow flower

½ ounce echinacea root

Mix the herbs in a bowl and store in a glass jar. Make tea by the cup. Steep 1 or 2 teaspoons in 10 ounces of hot water, covered, for 10 minutes. Give 3 cups a day, sweetened with honey if desired.

# ≡ NERVOUSNESS ≡

Unwrapping children's emotions is a delicate thing, but being there for them in loving and supportive ways is a tremendous help along the way. Ensuring my kids and pediatric patients have tools to support themselves is important too. Showing them ways to care for themselves can teach them empowerment, which has a way of crossing over to other areas of their life.

## Nerve-Support Drops

*Have these on hand for times of stress, nervousness, or shyness.*

2 teaspoons catnip leaf

1 teaspoon lemon balm leaf

1 teaspoon skullcap leaf

1 teaspoon hawthorn berry

2 ounces vegetable glycerin

Put the herbs in a 2-ounce jar and add vegetable glycerin to fill. Close tightly and shake well. Keep in a pantry or cupboard for 3 weeks, shaking every day. Strain and transfer to a 2-ounce dropper bottle. Give 5 drops to 1 dropperful as needed.

## Courage Drops

*Use these flower essence drops at times of anxiety, nervousness, or lack of confidence.*

4 drops crabapple flower essence

4 drops mimulus flower essence

4 drops aspen flower essence

4 drops walnut flower essence

1 ounce distilled water

5 milliliters brandy

Fill a 1-ounce dropper bottle with distilled water and add brandy for preservation. Add the flower essences and gently shake. Give 4 drops 4 times a day.

Nosebleeds are quite common in children, and most of the time they will grow out of them. As long as they have seen your health care provider to ensure there is not an underlying health condition, you can use the following recipes to manage until the vasculature further develops. Always do your best to keep your kiddo hydrated and ensure nasal tissues don't dry out.

## Healthy-Nose Tea

2 ounces peppermint leaf

1 ounce holy basil leaf

1 ounce yarrow leaf and flower

Mix the herbs in a bowl and store in a glass jar. Make tea by the pint. Add 3 tablespoons to a pint jar and pour boiling water over. Steep for 20 minutes. Give 4 ounces, 3 times a day to support healthy nasal tissues.

## Moist-Nose Oil

*Apply daily to prevent dryness and cracking of the nasal cavity.*

½ ounce yarrow leaf and flower

1 cup olive oil

40 drops coriander essential oil

10 drops peppermint essential oil

Put the herbs in a glass baking dish and cover with olive oil to a depth of 1 or 2 inches. Bake at 170 degrees F for 4 hours. Allow to cool and then strain. Pour into container of your choice and add the essential oils. Drip 3 to 4 drops onto a Q-tip and swab the inside of the nose as needed.

# ≡ SORE THROAT ≡

A sore throat can make the day hard to get through. When you've ruled out strep throat, these recipes will help to soothe the pain in the gentle way herbs do. But don't forget the good old-fashioned throat gargle using apple cider vinegar or warm water and salt. These traditional ways do the trick!

## Throat-Soothe Tea

2 ounces wild cherry bark

1 ounce marshmallow root

½ ounce licorice root

½ ounce thyme leaf

Mix the herbs in a bowl and store in a glass jar. Make tea by the cup. Steep 1 or 2 teaspoons in 10 ounces of hot water, covered, for 10 minutes. Give 3 cups a day until symptoms subside.

## Throat-Soothe Spray

2 teaspoons elderberry

2 teaspoons marshmallow root

½ teaspoon echinacea root

½ teaspoon ginger root

1 ounce apple cider vinegar

1 ounce vegetable glycerin

Put the herbs in a 2-ounce jar and add apple cider vinegar and vegetable glycerin to fill. Close tightly and shake well. Keep in a pantry or cupboard for 3 weeks, shaking every day. Strain and transfer to a 2-ounce spray bottle. Spray directly onto the throat multiple times a day.

## Throat-Soothe Oil

2 tablespoons chickweed leaf

2 tablespoons sage leaf

1 tablespoon cleavers leaf

¾ cup olive oil

Put the herbs in a glass baking dish and cover with olive oil to a depth of 1 or 2 inches. Bake at 170 degrees F for 4 hours. Allow to cool and then strain. Transfer to your bottle of your choice. Rub 1 teaspoon over external throat/neck area twice daily.

# ≡ TEA PARTY TIME ≡

I had no idea how much I'd enjoy tea parties once my child and I began having them. They were full-on affairs with tea, snacks, and fancy dress. I've always insisted on having real tea, because why not!

## Teatime Tea

2 ounces chamomile flower

¼ ounce ginger

¼ ounce licorice root

Mix the herbs in a bowl and store in a glass jar. Make tea by the cup. Steep 1 or 2 teaspoons in 10 ounces of hot water, covered, for 10 minutes.

## Lavender Cookies

*Nothing says tea party like little snacks. Having these on hand for your next tea party really raises the bar. This recipe makes about 6 dozen.*

½ cup butter, softened

½ cup shortening

1¼ cups sugar

2 large eggs

1 teaspoon vanilla extract

½ teaspoon almond extract

2¼ cups all-purpose flour

4 teaspoons dried lavender flower

1 teaspoon baking powder

½ teaspoon salt

Preheat oven to 375 degrees F. Cream the butter, shortening, and sugar until light and fluffy. Add the eggs, one at a time, beating well after each addition. Beat in the extracts. In a separate bowl, whisk the flour, lavender, baking powder, and salt; gradually beat into the creamed mixture. Drop by rounded teaspoonfuls 2 inches apart onto baking sheets lightly coated with cooking spray. Bake until golden brown, 8 to 10 minutes. Cool 2 minutes before removing to wire racks. Store in an airtight container.

My daughter seemed to sail through teething with little fuss. My son, on the other hand, seemed to always get two or three teeth at the same time. His fingers were perpetually in his mouth as he tried to comfort himself with something to bite on.

## Gum-Numbing Oil

*Combining olive oil with clove essential oil can help to numb the discomfort.*

2 ounces olive oil
15 drops clove essential oil

Mix together and keep in a jar. Dip a Q-tip into the oil and rub onto the gums when needed.

## Gum-Calming Tea

2 ounces chamomile flower
1 ounce lemon balm leaf

½ ounce catnip leaf
½ ounce oatstraw leaf

Mix the herbs in a bowl and store in a glass jar. Make tea by the cup. Steep 1 or 2 teaspoons in 10 ounces of hot water, covered, for 10 minutes. Offer teaspoon doses.

## CHAMOMILE PACIFIER MARINADE

Try soaking chamomile flowers in vegetable glycerin for 2 weeks, straining, and dipping a pacifer in it to offer to baby for comfort. You can also use this as a calming agent by applying to the gums with a clean finger or Q-tip.

# ≡ VACCINATION SUPPORT ≡

As our modern world advances and the schedule of recommended vaccinations continues to change, we must examine what is safe for our children. I am neither pro-vaccine nor anti-vaccine. I know the value and importance of vaccines yet do not agree with the recommended schedule. Young immune systems are just that—young. Vaccines are foreign substances that must be processed. Ensuring the body is capable of doing so is important before they are administered.

## Vaccine-Support Drops

2 teaspoons echinacea root

1 teaspoon chamomile flower

1 teaspoon hawthorn berry

1 teaspoon fennel seed

2 ounces vegetable glycerin

Put the herbs in a 2-ounce jar and pour glycerin over them until you fill the jar. Close tightly and shake well. Keep in a pantry or cupboard for 3 weeks, shaking every day. Strain and transfer to a 2-ounce dropper bottle. Give 1 dropperful 3 times a day for the 2 days before the vaccination and the 2 days after.

## Prevaccination-Support Powder

½ ounce elderberry powder

¼ ounce rosehips powder

¼ ounce ashwagandha powder

¼ ounce catnip powder

¼ ounce spirulina powder

Mix the powders in a bowl and store in a glass jar. Give ¼ teaspoon twice daily for 2 weeks before vaccinations.

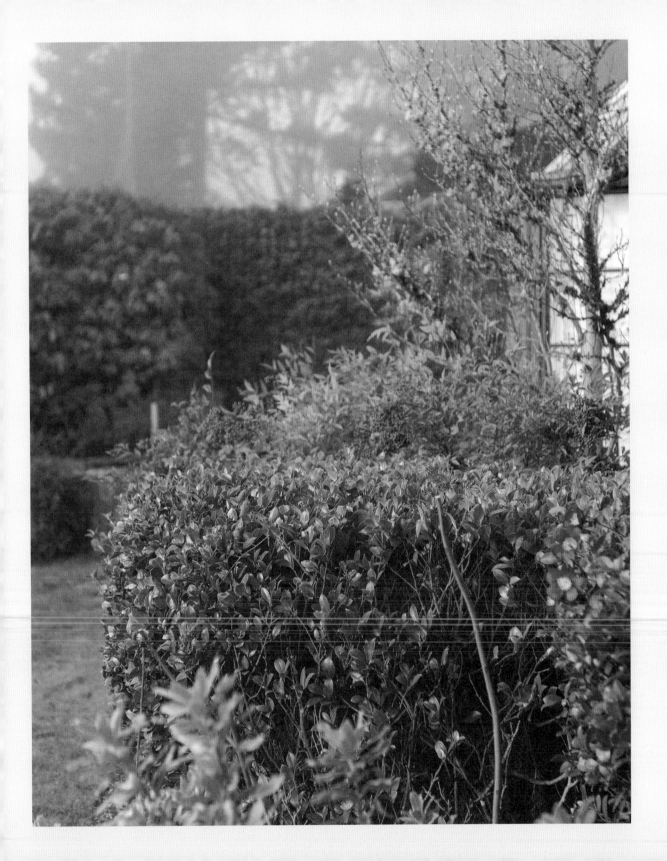

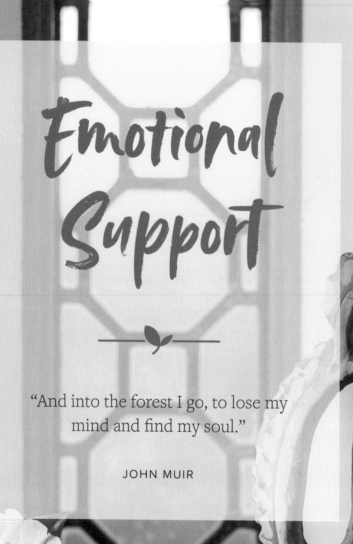

# Emotional Support

"And into the forest I go, to lose my mind and find my soul."

JOHN MUIR

AS OUR WORLD GROWS BIGGER AND BIGGER and as things seem to be spinning faster and faster, our emotional bodies are definitely affected. The ability to access our emotions is not something that is readily taught, but it should be. Navigating life takes skills, including learning to identify our feelings, knowing when we need help, and communicating our needs. Help can come from another person or through self-care. When I get overwhelmed—whether by work, my kids, or self-imposed pressure—I can now readily identify the physical feeling of stress and anxiety, and I know I need a time-out to make a cup of tea. Granted, it isn't always the most opportune time to take a moment out, but as a commitment to myself, I do. If I don't, I'll just keep going, and that feeling will get bigger and bigger and I'll start doing and saying things that are originating from that anxiety and stress versus from my authentic self.

When I make a cup of tea, I have to pause. It takes about 3 minutes to boil the water, and I give myself permission to just sit and wait and breathe. This creates the first shift for me to gain some perspective on whatever has triggered me. And then there is something about pouring the hot water over the herbs that really helps. It's like a hot waterfall, and my anxiety washes away with each splash of water. Dunking my herbs into and out of the water for a few minutes while the tea steeps becomes a meditation for me, and this action, combined with the aroma rising from the mug, deeply relaxes me. Sometimes the peace I get from this cup of tea lasts 5 hours, sometimes 5 minutes, but the commitment to doing it always reminds me to love and care for myself and those around me when emotions rise up.

So how do we learn to identify emotions? It is a slow, dedicated practice called awareness. This learning can be achieved through reading books, seeking professional guidance, meditation, exercise, journaling, or simply paying attention. When I first talk to patients about this practice, I remind them that awareness of emotions and patternistic behavior is a full-time job. When you begin, and then get better at it, you might notice that you feel anxious or irritated more than a hundred times a day, yet until now you weren't tuned in. Tuning in gives you the foundation to then seek out what is causing the feeling—and then ideally to shift it to move toward joy and peace.

When we work with emotional balance in herbal medicine, we often focus on the group of herbs called the nervines. Nervines are the herbs that work to protect, nourish, stimulate, or relax the central nervous system. Along with nervines, we also consider liver and digestive herbs to support the natural detoxification pathways and ensure metabolic by-products are not building up. Last, adaptogen herbs are important to support the stress-response centers of the body and ensure excess depletion stops and support is initiated.

Anxiety, depression, and any other emotional burden should be discussed with someone close to you. Living with the daily struggle of emotional imbalance can lead to feelings of isolation, fear, and hopelessness—none of which anyone deserves. We all struggle in this life in different ways. Having someone, anyone, remind us that we are not alone can create enough strength to keep going. Seek out community groups, free clinics, online resources, friends, and family for support. The first step is identifying the problem, but the hardest step is asking for help. May the herbs offer support for your peace of mind and guidance to begin living in balance with yourself.

## ═ ANXIETY ═

Anxiety appears for many different reasons. It can stem from trauma, medications, self-confidence issues, a physical disorder, or even allergic reactions to certain foods. It is characterized by a state of uneasiness and/or apprehension, and the reason for such concern may or may not be known.

## Nervine-Tonic Tea

*Drink this tea for general support of the central nervous system.*

1 ounce skullcap leaf

½ ounce agrimony leaf

½ ounce catnip leaf

½ ounce oatstraw

½ ounce lemon balm leaf

¾ ounce lemongrass

¼ ounce ginger root

Mix the herbs in a bowl and store in a glass jar. When needed, put 4 or 5 tablespoons in a quart jar and pour boiling water over the herbs to fill the jar. Let steep overnight and strain in the morning. Drink 2 to 3 cups a day for 8 to 12 weeks.

# Anxiety-Reduction Tincture

*This tincture can help reduce automatic nervous response and generalized anxiety.*

2 teaspoons lemon balm leaf

½ teaspoon schisandra berry

½ teaspoon celery seed

½ teaspoon chamomile flower

½ teaspoon oatstraw

2 ounces vodka

Put the herbs in a 2-ounce jar and add vodka to fill. Close tightly and shake well. Keep in a pantry or cupboard for 3 weeks, shaking every day. Strain and transfer to a 2-ounce dropper bottle. Take 1 dropperful 3 times a day.

# Anxiety-Calming Oil Blend

3 milliliters chamomile essential oil

1 milliliter frankincense essential oil

1 milliliter sweet orange essential oil

Pour the essential oils into a 5-milliliter bottle and gently shake. Carry it around with you so you can put a drop or two onto a handkerchief and inhale as needed for calming support.

# Nerve-Steadying Spritz

*When nerves are getting the best of you, use this spray. Nervousness is often centered around performance of a task or speaking up for oneself or in front of others.*

2 teaspoons hawthorn berry

1 teaspoon ginkgo leaf

¼ teaspoon hops strobiles

¾ teaspoon California poppy

2 ounces vodka

2 ounces vegetable glycerin

50 drops peppermint essential oil

Put the herbs in a 2-ounce jar and add vodka to fill. Close tightly and shake well. Keep in a pantry or cupboard for 3 weeks, shaking every day. Strain and transfer to a 4-ounce spray bottle. Add the vegetable glycerin and essential oil. Give yourself 1 or 2 spritzes under the tongue.

# ≡ DEPRESSION ≡

Depression, whether situational or long-standing, should always be discussed with a health care professional. It can be your family doctor, acupuncturist, counselor, or any other provider you feel comfortable with. Suffering alone can lead to hopelessness, which has a way of tricking the mind into thinking there is no way out. There is always a way out; it just sometimes takes longer to find the right support.

St. John's wort has been one of the most marketed herbs of late. While it originally was used to support nerve tissue and heal nerve damage, researchers and product companies alike have jumped on the bandwagon touting its supreme effects to lift mood and heal depression. The problem with that is that anytime an herb is marketed to such an extent, misinformation occurs and the herb itself often becomes pigeonholed for only one use. I use St. John's wort a lot, and yes, I do use it to lift mood when necessary, but we should always understand an herb's full potential and give credit where credit is due.

## Lift-My-Spirits Tea

*Make this tea when feelings of depression are slipping in and a mood shift is needed.*

1 ounce lemon balm leaf

1 ounce skullcap leaf

1 ounce orange peel

½ ounce St. John's wort leaf and flower

¼ ounce damiana leaf

¼ ounce hibiscus flower

Mix the herbs in a bowl and store in a glass jar. Make tea by the cup. Steep 1 or 2 teaspoons in 10 ounces of hot water, covered, for 10 minutes. Drink as needed.

# Positivity Tonic

1 ounce eleuthero root

1 ounce peppermint leaf

½ ounce ginkgo leaf

½ ounce hawthorne berry

½ ounce chamomile flower

½ ounce St. John's wort leaf and flower

Mix the herbs in a bowl and store in a glass jar. Make tea by the cup. Steep 1 teaspoon in 10 ounces of hot water, covered, for 10 minutes. Drink as needed.

# Happiness Balm

*This salve is a go-to when you need to remember that life is good in the midst of feeling not so good.*

2 tablespoons skullcap leaf

2 tablespoons chamomile flower

1 tablespoon lavender flower

¾ cup olive oil

½ ounce beeswax

40 drops clary sage essential oil

10 drops basil essential oil

10 drops lemon essential oil

Put the herbs in a glass baking dish and cover with olive oil to a depth of 1 or 2 inches. Bake at 170 degrees F for 4 hours. Allow to cool and then strain. Pour the oil into a saucepan and add the beeswax. Gently heat until the beeswax is melted. Pour into contaainer of your choice and add the essential oils. Rub a bit onto your temples and at the nape of your neck as needed.

# ≡ GRIEF ≡

Grief can come from losing something specific or from an internal place for unknown reasons. It is easy to identify when it comes from the loss of a person, pet, job, or special thing, but when there is no known cause it can be challenging to overcome and can often slide into depression. I typically turn to flower essences and homeopathy for grief, as they work so well to help process the emotion and allow us to move through it.

Ignatia is a homeopathic remedy specifically for grief, particularly when one hasn't been well since the passing of a loved one. Taking 5 pellets of a 30C Ignatia 3 times a day is something to consider when you are in this place. The flower essence borage helps relieve the deep weight of sorrow on our heart, and bleeding heart is great for those brokenhearted over the loss of someone or something.

## Grief-Relief Tea

1 ounce hawthorn berry

1 ounce chamomile flower

1 ounce linden flower

¾ ounce violet flower

¼ ounce licorice root

Mix the herbs in a bowl and store in a glass jar. Make tea by the cup. Steep 1 or 2 teaspoons in 10 ounces of hot water, covered, for 10 minutes. Drink as needed.

# ≡ PANIC ≡

Panic is the extreme result of anxiety. It often leads to physical symptoms of a racing heart, constricted breathing, sweating, hyperventilating, and sometimes passing out. It is a very out-of-control feeling. If you've sought treatment for your anxiety disorder and there is no overt health condition causing the disorder, herbs can help to sedate the sometimes intense feelings.

## Panic-Squelch Drops

*Take at the first sign of a panic attack.*

2 teaspoons California poppy

1 teaspoon black cohosh root

1 teaspoon hops strobiles

½ teaspoon passionflower leaf

½ teaspoon oatstraw

2 ounces vodka

Put the herbs in a 2-ounce jar and add vodka to fill. Close tightly and shake well. Keep in a pantry or cupboard for 3 weeks, shaking every day. Strain and transfer to a 2-ounce dropper bottle. Take 2 dropperfuls as needed.

## Quick-Shot Panic Relief

½ ounce kava tincture

1 ounce oatstraw tincture

Mix these two tinctures together in a shot glass and drink.

## Panic-Reduction Capsules

*These capsules promote healing of the central nervous system to reduce panic attacks.*

½ ounce passionflower leaf

½ ounce ashwagandha root

¼ ounce ginkgo leaf

¼ ounce St. John's wort leaf and flower

¼ ounce black cohosh root

¼ ounce holy basil leaf

Mix the powdered herbs in a bowl and fill 200 empty capsules. Take 2 capsules twice a day.

# Travel Wellness

—※—

"As the life of the horse is in his legs, so the life of the traveler is in his feet, and good care should be taken of them."

JULIETTE DE BAIRACLI LEVY

GETTING OUT TO EXPLORE THE WORLD offers insight into other cultures, yourself, and the diversity of life. When things feel stagnant or you've lost perspective, that's the time to travel. Whether you're taking off for someplace on the other side of the world or traveling just an hour or two by train, consider creating your own travel herbal medicine kit. If you eat the wrong thing or end up with an infected skin wound, having your herbal arsenal on hand will either take care of what you are dealing with or aid you until you can seek professional help. Being sick when you are traveling is never convenient, but having a well-curated travel kit can make a world of difference.

One example comes from a 2004 trip to Cuba I made with my boyfriend at the time, Dan. We ate a magnificent dinner near the end of the trip, each consuming different items, and by morning Dan was feverish and had severe stomach cramping. We were scheduled to leave the next morning but there was no way he was in traveling condition. What was I to do? I grabbed my herbal kit and first slathered castor oil onto his abdomen and gave him four herbal digestive capsules that I make specifically for traveling, to reduce cramping and kill bacteria. Next I rubbed an essential oil blend over his chest and feet. Then I made him a cup of yarrow tea and tucked him into bed. I repeated the capsules, tea, and oils every 2 hours. After about 3 hours he was able to sleep peacefully, and after about 6 hours he was returning to the land of the living.

## ≡ THE ESSENTIAL TRAVEL KIT ≡

I have this little kit ready to grab for getaways near and far. Recipes follow.

- Herbal Wound Spray
- Antibacterial Salve
- Lavender essential oil
- Digestion-Infection Capsules
- Traveler's-Tonic Drops

- Diarrhea-Stop Capsules
- Cold-Care Capsules
- Travel Cough Lozenges
- Immune-System-Up Drops
- Ma Huang Tincture

# Herbal Wound Spray

*Never ignore a tiny cut when traveling because you are being exposed to new and different bacteria perpetually. If a cut or scrape is red, streaking, swollen, tender, pus producing, or throbbing, treatment needs to be administered. Using a spray on a wound to clean it before applying a salve can greatly reduce the risk of infection.*

1 teaspoon calendula flower

1 teaspoon sage leaf

1 teaspoon yarrow leaf and flower

1 teaspoon goldenseal root

1 teaspoon myrrh resin

6 ounces hot water

½ ounce aloe vera juice

½ ounce witch hazel extract

sage essential oil

lavender essential oil

Steep the herbs in the hot water for 2 hours. Strain and put 1 ounce of the infusion in a 2-ounce spray bottle. Add the aloe vera juice, witch hazel extract, and essential oils. Gently shake to combine everything. Spray this onto a wound and dab with a cotton pad.

# Antibacterial Salve

*Having a salve to apply topically can serve a multitude of purposes. You can use it for cuts and scrapes to keep the area sealed off from infection, and you can also use it as lip balm or lip protector from strong weather elements.*

1 tablespoon calendula flower

1 tablespoon goldenseal root

½ tablespoon comfrey leaf

½ tablespoon lemon balm leaf

½ tablespoon chickweed leaf

½ tablespoon lavender flower

¾ cup olive oil

½ ounce beeswax

40 drops lemon essential oil

20 drops thyme essential oil

Put the herbs in a glass baking dish and cover with olive oil to a depth of 1 or 2 inches. Bake at 170 degrees F for 4 hours. Allow to cool and then strain. Pour the oil into a saucepan and add the beeswax. Gently heat until the beeswax is melted. Pour into container of your choice and add essential oils. Slather it on cuts and scrapes as needed.

## Digestion-Infection Capsules

*These are my go-to capsules when any stomach and/or lower digestive problem arises, whether caused by something you ate or water you drank or any of the many other things you might come into contact with when traveling.*

½ ounce cramp bark powder

¼ ounce Oregon grape root powder

¼ ounce valerian root powder

¼ ounce charcoal powder

¼ ounce goldenseal root powder

¼ ounce marshmallow root powder

⅛ ounce myrrh powder

⅛ ounce echinacea root powder

Mix the powdered herbs in a bowl and fill 200 empty capsules. Take 2 to 4 capsules every 2 hours until symptoms begin to subside. Then take 1 capsule 2 to 3 times a day for 7 days.

## THE INDISPENSABLE TRAVEL ESSENTIAL OIL: LAVENDER

I always have lavender essential oil with me when I travel. While traveling alone in Malta many years ago, I ended up camping on a beach for many days. I got a sunburn because I had no shade structure, and I also got a cut on my thumb while setting up my tent and ended up with about a thousand mosquito bites. Lavender quickly and efficiently healed each one of these troublesome issues. I put a few drops on my palms and rubbed my face, chest, and shoulders to relieve the sunburn heat. I put one drop directly onto the cut on my thumb, anticipating a sting, but nothing but instant soothing occurred. And last, I put drops on all of the mosquito-bitten regions of my body so I could finally get to sleep without the chronic itch.

Lavender is also extremely helpful with jetlag to help promote sleep and restfulness. I use it with my children on airplanes when they are anxious or overtired from a long day of traveling, and on myself when I'm reaching my wits' end. Experiencing a headache while traveling? Try rubbing a bit onto your temples or the nape of your neck.

# OTHER ESSENTIAL OILS FOR TRAVELING

- **CHAMOMILE:** for sleep

- **GERANIUM:** for dry skin and to help keep hormones in balance if traveling has thrown your menstrual cycle off track

- **GINGER:** for digestion and particularly for nausea

- **ORANGE** or **LEMON:** for when your hotel room isn't as fresh as you had expected and you need a few spritzes to clear the air

- **PEPPERMINT:** for upset stomachs, respiratory congestion, headache, fever, and sore muscles, and to give yourself some extra energy to get through the next flight

- **RAVENSARA:** to rub onto oneself if exposure is a concern

- **ROSE:** for stressful travel moments

- **TEA TREE:** to use as a hand sanitizer and for bug bites

## Traveler's-Tonic Drops

*I take these drops before each and every meal when I travel. It helps to protect against contamination but also against inability to digest new foods that my system doesn't quite know how to handle.*

2 teaspoons Oregon grape root

1 teaspoon triphala

1 teaspoon olive leaf

½ teaspoon ginger root

½ teaspoon fennel seed

2 ounces apple cider vinegar

Put the herbs in a 2-ounce jar and add apple cider vinegar to fill. Close tightly and shake well. Keep in a pantry or cupboard for 3 weeks, shaking every day. Strain and transfer to a 2-ounce dropper bottle. Take 1 dropperful before each meal.

## Diarrhea-Stop Capsules

*I typically recommend capsules for diarrhea because the medicine passes directly through the digestive system. That being said, this can easily be converted to drops if you prefer or are worried about too much elimination occurring for the medicine to get effectively broken down and utilized.*

½ ounce plantain leaf powder

½ ounce sage leaf powder

¼ ounce goldenseal root powder

¼ ounce raspberry leaf powder

¼ ounce slippery elm bark powder

¼ ounce echinacea root powder

Mix the powdered herbs in a bowl and fill 200 empty capsules. Take 2 capsules every 2 to 3 hours until symptoms subside.

## Cold-Care Capsules

*This general blend is to target basic cold symptoms of runny nose, congestion, and respiratory complaints.*

½ ounce myrrh powder

½ ounce yarrow leaf and flower powder

¼ ounce usnea lichen powder

¼ ounce lion's mane mushroom powder

¼ ounce horehound leaf powder

¼ ounce ginger root powder

Mix the powdered herbs in a bowl and fill 200 empty capsules. Take 2 capsules 4 times a day as needed.

## Travel Cough Lozenges

*Sitting on a plane with a cough is the worst. Having these lozenges to soothe the cough and boost your immune defenses will make you, and your neighbor, much happier.*

½ tablespoon horehound leaf

½ tablespoon sage leaf

½ tablespoon wild cherry bark

1 teaspoon ashwagandha root

1 teaspoon chamomile flower

¾ cup boiling water

¾ cup honey

5–10 drops sweet orange essential oil

slippery elm bark powder

Steep the herbs in the boiling water for 1 hour and then strain and pour into a small saucepan. Add the honey and heat over medium heat just until the mixture begins to boil.

Using a candy thermometer, determine when the temperature reaches 300 degrees F and then turn off the heat. Let the mixture cool for 5 to 10 minutes, until it starts to get syrupy. Add the essential oil. Drop by small spoonfuls onto parchment paper and let cool. Dust with slippery elm bark powder and once they are completely cooled, store in a glass jar. Melt in mouth as needed.

## Immune-System-Up Drops

*Before I get on a plane I take a dropperful of this blend to tell my immune system to be on the alert. You can also take this a couple of days before a trip, especially when you are traveling long distances and sleep will be compromised.*

2 teaspoons reishi mushroom

1 teaspoon ashwagandha root

1 teaspoon nettle leaf

½ teaspoon spirulina

½ teaspoon rosehips

2 ounces vodka

Put the herbs in a 2-ounce jar and add vodka to fill. Close tightly and shake well. Keep in a pantry or cupboard for 3 weeks, shaking every day. Strain and transfer to a 2-ounce dropper bottle. Take 1 dropperful right before plane, train, or bus travel.

## Ma Huang Tincture

*If you can get ahold of some ma huang (ephedra) and make a small amount of tincture it is another herb of value when traveling. Use it for breathing constriction or sudden allergic reaction until you can get professional medical attention.*

2 teaspoons ma huang

1 ounce vodka

Place ma huang in a 1-ounce jar and add vodka to fill. Close tightly and shake well. Keep in a pantry or cupboard for 3 weeks, shaking every day. Strain and transfer to a 2-ounce dropper bottle. Take 1 dropperful 3 times a day as needed.

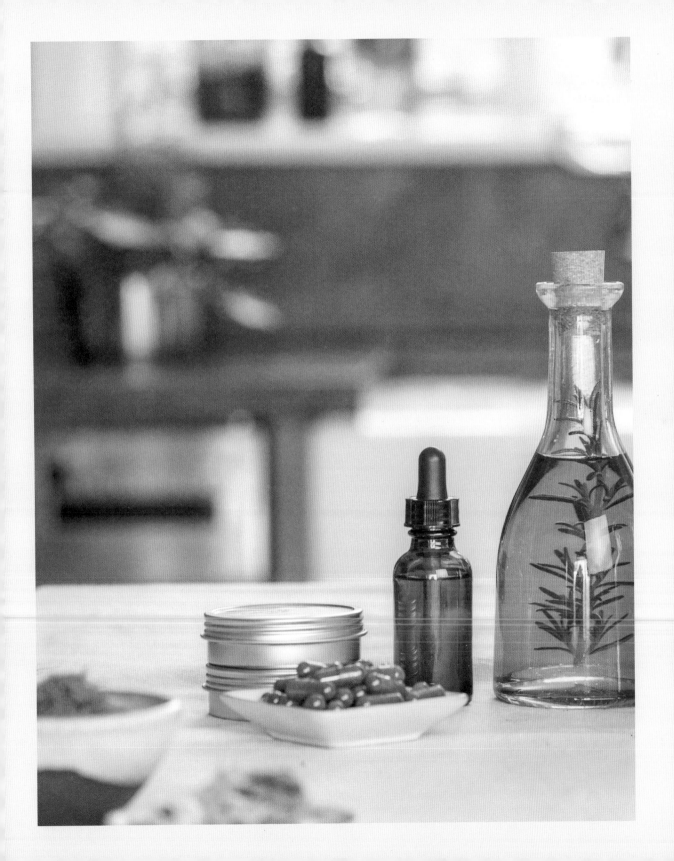

# Herbs for Elders

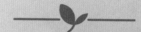

"The doctor of the future will give no medicine, but will interest his patients in the care of the human frame, in diet, and in the cause and prevention of disease."

THOMAS EDISON

TIME ELUDES NO ONE. While some are excellent at getting well, exercising regularly, and keeping stress down, most of us are just doing the best we can. No matter which category we fall in, our body ages as we age. The things enumerated in this section are common complaints I treat with my customers and patients. Caring for your body throughout your life is the best prevention, but even if you haven't, you don't have to suffer through the years. Herbs and other treatments can radically shift your body back to ease and comfort. No one can deny that movement is one of the best ways to keep the fluids of the body moving and the joints and systems lubricated. Movement also keeps blood moving to the brain and the digestive organs relaxed. And exercise liberates stored fat and hormones that help to maintain balance in bones and emotional well-being. Movement and relaxation techniques such as yoga are proven to reduce stress and also cholesterol.

Herbs, on the other hand, work to correct imbalances and shift physical processes back to health. Throughout the book we've seen them used for both acute and chronic problems. In my elder population I like to encourage daily use to nourish and tone the body. When you use them over a period of time you rebuild the systems so that symptoms are diminished and the organs work as they should.

## ⟩ ARTHRITIS ⟨

Arthritis by definition means inflamed joints. Over the years, the normal wear and tear on our joints begins to take a toll. Arthritis tends to start in one joint and can begin at any age. The story I typically hear is it started a year ago in one area and then slowly got worse and spread to other joints. When we are younger, we have a tendency to ignore our body's inconveniences, but treating them supports our body to be stronger as we age.

# Anti-Arthritis Capsules

*While healing arthritis is not common, you can reduce the discomforts and support the tissues from further damage by taking these capsules to provide relief from inflammation and swelling.*

½ ounce frankincense resin powder

½ ounce turmeric root powder

¼ ounce cat's claw powder

¼ ounce ginger powder

¼ ounce burdock root powder

¼ ounce yucca root powder

Mix the powdered herbs in a bowl and fill 200 empty capsules. Take 2 capsules twice a day.

# Herbal Icy Hot Rub

*Apply this salve to any joint for temporary cooling of arthritis discomfort.*

2 tablespoons white willow bark

1 tablespoon frankincense resin

2 teaspoons menthol crystals

1 teaspoon peppermint leaf

¾ cup olive oil

½ ounce beeswax

Put the herbs in a glass baking dish and cover with olive oil to a depth of 1 or 2 inches. Bake at 170 degrees F for 4 hours. Allow to cool and then strain. Pour the oil into a saucepan and add the beeswax. Gently heat until the beeswax is melted and then pour into container of your choice. Apply as needed to sore joints.

# Arthritis-Relief Castor Oil

*Using this infused castor oil should reduce discomfort, but it works on deeper levels than simply pain relief. A great anti-inflammatory, castor oil is absorbed through the skin and can lubricate the joint as well. It also stimulates the immune system to help if autoantibodies are part of the arthritis picture.*

2 tablespoons hydrangea root

1 tablespoon chaparral leaf

1 tablespoon black cohosh root

1 teaspoon lobelia leaf

¾ cup castor oil

Put the herbs in a glass baking dish and pour castor oil over the herbs to a depth of 1 or 2 inches. Bake at 170 degrees F for 4 hours. Allow to cool and then strain. Apply 1 or 2 teaspoons to the painful area and cover with a cotton towel and then a heating pad or hot water bottle.

# TIPS FOR PREVENTING AND EASING ARTHRITIS PAIN

- Add turmeric to your diet.

- Take Anti-Arthritis Capsules.

- Exercise.

- Meditate for pain management.

- Ensure you are drinking enough water to be properly hydrated.

- Get a massage or try acupuncture.

- Use hydrotherapy, alternating hot and cold water.

- Topically apply Arthritis-Relief Castor Oil packs.

## BLADDER CONTROL

Keeping the ligaments toned as we age helps many parts of our body stay strong and in their correct places. Bladder strength is often a problem as we age due to hormone imbalance and weakening of the muscles and the ligaments that support it. Increasing the tone of the pelvic floor muscles can help to reduce bladder weakness. Yoga is great for this, as are many floor exercises.

## Bladder-Tone Capsules

½ ounce reishi mushroom powder

½ ounce fo-ti powder

¼ ounce eleuthero root powder

¼ ounce goldenrod leaf powder

¼ ounce raspberry leaf powder

¼ ounce cornsilk powder

Mix the powdered herbs in a bowl and fill 200 empty capsules. Take 2 capsules twice a day.

# ≡ BRAIN SUPPORT ≡

Supporting the brain as we age is almost as important as exercise. While I subscribe to my mom's theory that crossword puzzles keep the mind sharp, I also think her active social life plays a big role. Having a community to share experiences with and to feel a part of helps keep us connected and involved in the world around us. We still can't get around the simple fact that aging affects the brain, but supporting it as we do the rest of the body can slow deterioration.

## Brain-Food Capsules

½ ounce rosemary leaf powder

½ ounce ginkgo leaf powder

¼ ounce eleuthero root powder

¼ ounce holy basil leaf powder

¼ ounce spirulina powder

¼ ounce hawthorn berry powder

Mix the powdered herbs in a bowl and fill 200 empty capsules. Take 1 or 2 capsules twice a day for a toning effect, or take as needed.

## Brain-Boost Blend

5 milliliters frankincense essential oil

2 milliliters lemon essential oil

2 milliliters lavender essential oil

1 milliliter vetiver essential oil

Blend the oils in a 10-milliliter essential oil bottle. Drop 1 or 2 drops into your palms, rub together, and take 3 deep inhalations. Alternatively you can add 5 drops to your room diffuser.

# ≡ COLDNESS AND CIRCULATION ≡

My mother is always cold. Each year we go on a family camping trip in the Pacific Northwest, where camping trips are often on the damp and chilly side, and I'm perpetually worried she'll be too chilled to enjoy herself. They say blood thickens as we age, which can slow circulation. We also tend to hold more blood in our core as we age to support the heart. Again, exercise is important here. If you suffer from feeling cold all the time, testing should be done to ensure that body temperature regulating systems like the thyroid are okay, and if everything comes back normal you can move on to considering herbal circulatory support.

## Body-Warming Drops

*Using a little herb called lobelia can be just the thing to get blood moving all the way down to our fingertips and toes.*

2 teaspoons ginkgo leaf

1 teaspoon prickly ash bark

½ teaspoon ginger root

¼ teaspoon lobelia leaf

¹⁄₁₆ teaspoon cayenne powder

2 ounces vodka

Put the herbs in a 2-ounce jar and add vodka to fill. Close tightly and shake well. Keep in a pantry or cupboard for 3 weeks, shaking every day. Strain and transfer to a 2-ounce dropper bottle. Take 1 dropperful as needed to increase internal warmth.

## Warming Hand-and-Foot Rub

*Take time out by the fire to rub on this warming balm. Better yet, get someone to give you a foot rub with it.*

2 tablespoons thyme leaf

1 tablespoon rosemary leaf

1 tablespoon ginger root

¾ cup olive oil

½ ounce beeswax

20 drops black pepper essential oil

Put the herbs in a glass baking dish and cover with olive oil to a depth of 1 or 2 inches. Bake at 170 degrees F for 4 hours. Allow to cool and then strain. Pour the oil into a saucepan and add the beeswax. Gently heat until the beeswax is melted. Pour into container of your choice and add essential oil. Apply as needed.

## Circulatory-Pizzazz Capsules

*Want to increase circulation in general to get the blood moving? Try these. Wear gloves to make them, due to the cayenne powder.*

½ ounce turmeric root powder

½ ounce panax ginseng powder

½ ounce ginkgo leaf powder

¼ ounce prickly ash bark powder

¼ ounce parsley leaf powder

⅛ teaspoon cayenne pepper powder

Mix the powdered herbs in a bowl and fill 200 empty capsules. Take 2 capsules once or twice daily.

# ═ INSOMNIA AND FITFUL SLEEP ═

This is another one of those nuisances that strikes many of us as we age. See "Insomnia" in the "Day-to-Day Health" section for recommendations.

# ═ MUSCLE SORENESS AND STIFFNESS ═

Whether it's from sitting too long or from overworking in the yard, stiffness has a way of settling into older bones and muscles. Drink plenty of water to ensure lactic acid doesn't build up, consider taking a magnesium powder to help the muscles relax, and check out the herbal recipes here for further support.

## Gardening-Ease Tea

*Drink this throughout your gardening time to help reduce muscle inflammation and future discomfort.*

1 ounce alfalfa leaf

1 ounce nettle leaf

¾ ounce hibiscus flower

½ ounce comfrey leaf

½ ounce lemon balm leaf

¼ ounce ginger root

Mix the herbs in a bowl and store in a glass jar. Make tea by the cup. Steep 1 or 2 teaspoons in 10 ounces of hot water, covered, for 10 minutes. Sip during gardening.

## Ache-Ease Herbal Bath Salts

*Add these to a hot bath after doing strenuous work.*

16 ounces Epsom salt

8 ounces Dead Sea salt

100 drops lavender essential oil

60 drops clary sage essential oil

40 drops cypress essential oil

Add everything to a large ziplock bag and shake well. Store in a glass jar and use as needed, 1 to 2 cups per bath.

## Sore-Muscle Rub

Poplar is one of my favorite herbs for sore muscles. Around late January or early February if you live where poplar grows, consider checking the trees for buds. If you see them, or most likely smell them (they have a lovely scent), begin looking for fallen limbs to collect the buds. Gather a handful or two and take them home to process. Put them in a pan you don't want to reuse and add enough olive oil to cover the fresh buds to a depth of 1 to 2 inches. Bake in the oven at 170 degrees F for 2 or 3 days. Your home will smell incredible and then you can strain the oil into a bottle of your choice. Apply a bit to anything that hurts for a magical melting away of pain and discomfort. Want to skip the work? Contact your local herb shop to purchase the oil already prepared.

## ≡ VISION CHANGES ≡

Vision changes are happening earlier and earlier in life with the use of computers and smart phones. Using the tea and syrup here, along with eye exercises, can greatly help.

## Eye-Strengthener Tea

1 ounce bilberry

1 ounce rooibos leaf

½ ounce turmeric root

½ ounce vanilla powder

¼ ounce calendula flower

¼ ounce yellow dock root

¼ ounce cinnamon chips

⅛ ounce whole cloves

⅛ ounce cardamom pods

Mix the herbs in a bowl and store in a glass jar. Make tea by the cup. Steep 1 or 2 teaspoons in 10 ounces of water, covered, for 10 minutes. Add coconut or hemp milk if you prefer a creamer drink. Drink 1 to 2 cups a day for 4 to 8 weeks.

## Eye-Strengthener Syrup

1 ounce eyebright leaves and stems

1 ounce bilberry

½ ounce hawthorn berry

½ ounce hawthorn leaf and flower

½ ounce horse chestnut

½ ounce ginkgo leaf

8 cups water

3 cups cane sugar or honey

¼ cup apple cider vinegar

Put the herbs in a saucepan with the water, bring to a boil, and reduce by half on medium-low heat. Strain the herbs out and put the brew back into the pan. Add sugar or honey and gently heat to mix if necessary, stirring continously. Turn off the heat, add the apple cider vinegar, and allow to cool. Then transfer to container of your choice and store in the refrigerator. Take 1 teaspoon once or twice daily.

## Weepy Eyes

While infection, irritation, allergies, and other causes for watery eyes exist, one of the most common causes of watery eyes and tearing is dry eyes. From the Chinese medicine perspective, we also have to consider a kidney deficiency as the kidneys are responsible for the waterways of the body and the kidneys tend to diminish in health as we age. The homeopathic remedy Natrum Muraticum is often a very effective treatment for weepy eyes.

## Eye-Hydration Tea

1 ounce alfalfa leaf

1 ounce rosehips

¾ ounce raspberry leaf

½ ounce chamomile flower

½ ounce peppermint leaf

¼ ounce ginger root

Mix the herbs in a bowl and store in a glass jar. When needed, steep 4 or 5 tablespoons in a quart of hot water. Drink 3 cups a day for 4 to 6 weeks.

## Eye-Support Drops

*This formula focuses on the problem arising from a weakness in the kidneys or liver.*

2 teaspoons fo-ti root

1 teaspoon burdock root

1 teaspoon bupleurum root

1 teaspoon hydrangea root

2 ounces vodka

Put the herbs in a 2-ounce jar and add vodka to fill. Close tightly and shake well. Keep in a pantry or cupboard for 3 weeks, shaking every day. Strain and transfer to a 2-ounce dropper bottle. Take 1 dropperful 3 times a day for 3 to 6 weeks.

## EXERCISES FOR BETTER VISION

- Sit with the head still and facing forward. Look to the left and focus on what you see. Then look to the right and focus on what you see. Do the same looking up and then looking down, all without moving your head. Repeat this 3 times.

- Imagine a giant figure 8 in front of you on the floor. Trace the shape with your eyes for a few minutes and then trace it in the reverse direction for a few mintues.

- Hold your thumb out as far in front of you as your arm will reach and focus on it. Then bring it within a few inches of your face and focus again. Do this 5 times.

- Find somewhere outside to sit and find three objects, one that is 50 feet away, one that is 20 feet away, and one that is 5 feet away. Look and focus on each one in succession for 30 seconds. Repeat this 5 times.

# Herbs for Odds and Ends

"The next major advance in the health of the
American people will be determined by what the
individual is willing to do for himself."

JOHN KNOWLES

WE OFTEN THINK OF HERBS as being used only for health and healing, but they have been used in many other ways as well. To wrap up this book I wanted to include a random collection of recipes that I find helpful and fun—for animal care, natural dyeing, and making scented notepaper, to name just a couple. As a do-it-yourselfer and explorer, I've collected these recipes over many years.

## ═ ANIMAL CARE ═

Another passion of mine is animals. I've always had a soft spot in my heart for animals, having had pets and worked with animals most of my life. Recently we were visiting with family and they asked my daughter how many animals we had. Despite being engaged in another conversation, I about fell out of my chair when she replied that we had thirty-three animals. Somehow my love has grown into an animal addiction! The alpaca is going to have to wait, especially since a week later one of our dogs had her puppies. But I digress. Having the skills to care for my loved ones of every species means I save money as well as provide them with top-notch care.

## Flea Repellent Oil

*Natural flea care can be successful, but diligence is necessary. As with anything, prevention is key, but consistent treatment can eradicate the problem if it occurs.*

10 drops rosemary essential oil

5 drops peppermint essential oil

5 drops eucalyptus essential oil

5 drops tea tree essential oil

5 drops citronella essential oil

1 ounce jojoba oil

3 ounces witch hazel extract

Blend the ingredients in a 4-ounce spray bottle and gently shake. Spray on pet's coat daily during high season and every 1 to 3 days during low season. Be sure to also spray on the animal's collar and bedding.

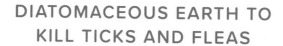

# DIATOMACEOUS EARTH TO KILL TICKS AND FLEAS

Food-grade diatomaceous earth has long been used to kill fleas and ticks. It works by cutting their exoskeleton (their hard outer shell) and then sucking the water out of their bodies. While some pet owners are comfortable putting it directly onto their animal's fur, I think it has the tendency to dry out the coat and cause itchiness. Better to use it on bedding, your yard, or your carpet. Begin by combing the area with a broom or rake. This agitates the fleas and gets them moving. Then sprinkle the diatomaceous earth on the area. For carpet, wait 12 hours before vacuuming. Repeat once a week for 4 weeks to ensure all eggs have completed their life cycle and no adults remain to lay more eggs.

## Herbal Flea Powder

*Some animals are fearful of the spray sound and feeling. In these cases a powder may be better. They may also attach to the fur shaft better.*

1 cup arrowroot powder

20 drops rosemary essential oil

20 drops wintergreen essential oil

10 drops eucalyptus essential oil

10 drops citronella essential oil

Mix the ingredients and store in a glass shaker bottle. Gently rub the powder into the fur every few days during high season. Be sure to sprinkle some on the animal's bedding.

## Coat-Health Formula

*If a pet's coat is dull, usually there is a food allergy or mineral deficiency causing the problem. Adding an herbal powder to the pet's food can dramatically improve coat health. Most animals—dogs, goats, chickens, ducks, alpacas, what have you—will eat it no matter what*

262

*you put it on. Cats, on the other hand, can be finicky. But the kelp is a little fishy and I've found most cats like it. Adding a little bit of tuna juice can help too.*

**1 ounce nettle leaf powder**          **1 ounce spirulina powder**

**1 ounce alfalfa leaf powder**          **1 ounce kelp powder**

Mix the ingredients in a bowl and store in a glass jar. Add to food according to pet's weight.

4–15 pounds: ¼ teaspoon twice daily

16–30 pounds: 1 teaspoon twice daily

31–50 pounds: 2 teaspoons twice daily

51 pounds and up: 1 tablespoon twice daily

## Deworming Formula

If worms are a problem, use the Coat-Health Formula but add ½ ounce wormwood powder and ¼ ounce black walnut hull powder. Give the same dosage.

## ≡ NATURAL DYEING ≡

Using plants to dye fabrics and fibers is certainly not easier than using commercial dyes, but it is much more rewarding. The colors that result are beautifully subdued and often take on the scent of the plant used.

Two basic types of fibers are used in dyeing. The first type has higher protein content and is often of animal origin such as wool and silk. The second type is plant-based fibers such as cotton and linen that are cellulose based. Protein-based fibers tend to take on dye much easier than plant-based fibers, but using a mordant (a substance that combines with the dye to make it fix to the fabric better) helps. Typically used mordants are alum, chrome, tin, iron, copper sulphate, and cream of tartar.

Another thing to consider is if the plant dye is more alkaline or more acidic. This helps you determine how it will wash. A more alkaline dye will wash better than a more acidic dye because most soaps are also alkaline. To make the dye, you use roughly 1 ounce of plant material to 32 ounces of water. Typically you boil the water with the plant material to reach the color desired and then strain. You then submerge the fabric or fiber in the dyed water, spreading it out for soaking to get a consistent color.

# HERBS FOR NATURAL DYEING

Some of the following chart was taken from *The Encyclopedia of Herbs and Herbalism* by Malcolm Stuart.

| Color | Herb | Mordant |
|---|---|---|
| gray | horsetail leaf | alum |
| light golden brown | flax seed | tin and cream of tartar |
| orange | tansy flower | chrome and cream of tartar |
| clear yellow | calendula flower, carrot | alum |
| creamy yellow | birch bark | alum |
| soft blue/lavender | elderberry | none or alum and salt |
| purple | dandelion root | tin and vinegar |
| red | St. John's wort flower | tin |
| rusty red | cleavers leaf | none |
| magenta | dandelion root | alum |
| orange-yellow | turmeric root | none needed |
| red-pink | hibiscus flower | none needed |
| gray-black | sumac leaf, meadowsweet leaf | none needed |

The following recipes are an eclectic group that remind me of another time.

## Thyme to Clean

*I don't know about you, but I rarely whistle while I work. But this formula does put a smile on my face at how well it cleans and disinfects!*

peels from 2 lemons

2 small bunches of fresh thyme sprigs

2 cups distilled white vinegar

1 tablespoon castile soap

2 cups water

100 drops lemon essential oil

Put the lemon peels and thyme into a pint mason jar with the vinegar. Close and let steep for 2 weeks, shaking daily. Strain and pour half into a 24-ounce spray bottle. Add the castile soap, water, and essential oil. Shake before use. Apply to a cloth and clean away.

## Rose-Petal Sink Scrubber

*This is a powerful cleaner with a delicate touch. Cleaning the sink is one of my least favorite jobs but seeing it shine afterward is worth the work.*

½ cup baking soda

½ cup borax

½ cup ground rose petals

½ cup fine kosher or sea salt

15 drops rose essential oil

Combine the ingredients in a glass jar with a sprinkle top for easy use. Sprinkle the mixture all over the sink, add a drop or two of dish soap to your cleaning sponge or brush, and get at it.

# Lavender Carpet Cleaner

*Relax! This carpet cleaner will pull out bad odors and create a sense of calm in your household. Don't care for lavender? Use your preferred essential oil.*

2 cups baking soda
60–100 drops lavender essential oil

Combine the ingredients in a glass jar and sprinkle all over the carpet when ready to use. Allow the mixture to sit on the carpet for at least 20 minutes before vacuuming up. Add 2 cups diatomaceous earth if you are concerned about fleas.

# Lemon Glass Cleaner

*Warning! Small children, animals, and my husband have been known to run into glass doors cleaned with this product because it works so well.*

1 ounce lemongrass
2 cups apple cider vinegar
2 tablespoons distilled water
20 drops lemon essential oil

Put the lemongrass into a pint mason jar with the vinegar. Close and let steep for 2 weeks, shaking daily. Strain and pour into a spray bottle. Add the distilled water and essential oil. If you have hard-core goop on your windows, add 1 tablespoon cream of tartar for stain-fighting power. Spray it on the glass and let it sit for a few minutes before wiping clean.

# Fly Repellent

*Use this spray to help keep the flies away. Tansy works great, but some have sensitivity to it.*

2 tablespoons fresh tansy flower
1 tablespoon fresh lavender flower
1 tablespoon fresh rosemary leaf
1 tablespoon fresh peppermint leaf
1 cup witch hazel extract
20 drops essential oil of your choice
   (I use lavender and lemon)

Steep the herbs in 1 cup of hot water, covered, for 1 hour. Strain, add the witch hazel and essential oil, and put into a spray bottle. Spritz as needed.

# Air Sweeteners

*Scent sprays are among my favorite things. They are easy to make, and scent is such a simple pleasure. Just one spritz and I can be transformed. Don't go buy a bunch of essential oils—use what you have either alone or in combination. Here are four of my favorite recipes.*

Put all the ingredients in a 2-ounce spray bottle and shake before use.

### BATHROOM BLISS

2 ounces distilled water

15 drops lemon essential oil

10 drops orange essential oil

5 drops bergamot essential oil

### BEDTIME SPRITZ

2 ounces distilled water

15 drops lavender essential oil

5 drops frankincense essential oil

2 drops vetiver essential oil

### VANILLA ROOM SPRAY

2 ounces witch hazel extract

15 drops vanilla essential oil

2 drops orange essential oil

### SPRING DAY SPRAY

2 ounces distilled water

15 drops neroli essential oil

7 drops jasmine essential oil

3 drops lime essential oil

# Potpourri

*You may believe that potpourri was just a fad, but having these scented herbs in the open airways of your home can not only promote energy, relaxation, or focus but also combat winter colds and flus. Choose a pretty bowl and set it out for display. The volatile oils will waft into the air, but stick your hands in it and rub them together before taking a nice big inhalation. Alternatively you can make simmering potpourri. This is simply adding the ingredients to a simmer pot on the stove.*

### CHAI SIMMERING POTPOURRI

4 black tea bags

1 teaspoon whole cloves

1 teaspoon nutmeg

1 teaspoon cardamom

1 teaspoon ginger

1 teaspoon cinnamon chips

6 cups water

Add all ingredients to a saucepan or simmer pot and simmer on very low.

### FOCUS SIMMERING POTPOURRI

6–8 sprigs fresh rosemary

4 sprigs fresh thyme

1 sprig fresh sage

peel of 1 lemon

6 cups water

Add all ingredients to a saucepan or simmer pot and simmer on very low.

### GERM-BLASTER POTPOURRI

2 handfuls of each of the following:
  lavender, cedar, bitter orange
  peel, lemon balm, hibiscus, juniper
  berries, star anise, and rose petals

1–2 tablespoons orris root powder

10 drops spruce essential oil

5 drops clove essential oil

5 drops ginger essential oil

5 drops lemon essential oil

Mix the herbs in a bowl with the orris root powder and essential oils. Put into an airtight container for 1 to 2 weeks to allow to set, and then it's ready to go!

## HERB PILLOWS

Just a little pouch of herbs can pack a powerful punch. Some people carry around essential oils, but I carry around herb pillows. They are typically 3 inches by 4 inches but can be made larger or smaller. Choose your fabric, stitch it up, and pack it full of herbs. Try these combinations to get started.

- ❧ SLEEP: lavender, hops, chamomile, roses, skullcap, mugwort, sandalwood, cedar
- ❧ BRAIN STIMULATION: rosemary, peppermint, frankincense, lemon, pine, basil
- ❧ MEDITATION: myrrh, sage, rosemary, Atlas cedar, rose
- ❧ MOTH REPELLANT: bay, cinnamon, cedar, thyme, rosemary, lemon peel, clove

## TUSSIE-MUSSIES

I adore tussie-mussies. These miniature arrangements of herbs and flowers share with us the secret language of plants. "Tussie-mussie" originates from the Victorian era and means a small, round bouquet of herbs and flowers with symbolic meanings. Making one simply requires you to know which plants mean what and to arrange a bouquet. Here is a snippet.

- ❧ GRASS: alludes to the fleeting quality of life
- ❧ WHITE ROSEBUD: a heart untouched by love
- ❧ ELDERBERRY: sympathy
- ❧ WOOD SORREL: maternal love
- ❧ GOLDENROD: encouragement
- ❧ FLOWERING REED: confidence in heaven
- ❧ OPIUM POPPY: forgetfulness
- ❧ ROSEMARY: remembrance
- ❧ COLTSFOOT: justice shall be done you

## SCENTED NOTEPAPER

While it may have been a while since you've handwritten a letter, I still cherish the experience. I have special paper and find quietness in sharing thoughts with a friend this way. I often fill a Tupperware box with a few sheets of paper and a piece of tissue with 10 drops of essential oil. I let it infuse the paper for a couple of days. The scent depends on who I'm writing to, but I do have a signature scent, rich in exotic remembrance.

# METRIC CONVERSIONS

| Inches | Centimeters |
|--------|-------------|
| 1 | 2.5 |
| 2 | 5.0 |
| 5 | 12.7 |

| Feet | Meters |
|------|--------|
| 1 | 0.3 |
| 2 | 0.6 |
| 3 | 0.9 |
| 4 | 1.2 |
| 5 | 1.5 |
| 10 | 3.0 |
| 50 | 15.2 |
| 100 | 30.5 |

| US Volume Measure | Metric Equivalent |
|-------------------|-------------------|
| ⅟₁₆ teaspoon | 0.3 milliliter |
| ⅛ teaspoon | 0.5 milliliter |
| ¼ teaspoon | 1.2 milliliters |
| ½ teaspoon | 2.5 milliliters |
| 1 teaspoon | 5.0 milliliters |
| 1 tablespoon (3 teaspoons) | 14.8 milliliters |
| 2 tablespoons (1 fluid ounce) | 29.6 milliliters |
| ⅛ cup (2 tablespoons) | 29.6 milliliters |
| ¼ cup (4 tablespoons) | 59.1 milliliters |
| ½ cup (4 fluid ounces) | 118.3 milliliters |
| ¾ cup (6 fluid ounces) | 177.4 milliliters |
| 1 cup (16 tablespoons) | 236.6 milliliters |
| 1 pint (2 cups) | 473.2 milliliters |
| 1 quart (4 cups) | 946.4 milliliters |

| US Weight Measure | Metric Equivalent |
|-------------------|-------------------|
| ⅟₁₆ ounce | 1.8 grams |
| ⅛ ounce | 3.5 grams |
| ¼ ounce | 7.0 grams |
| ½ ounce | 14.2 grams |
| ¾ ounce | 21.3 grams |
| 1 ounce | 28.3 grams |
| 1½ ounces | 42.5 grams |
| 2 ounces | 56.7 grams |
| 3 ounces | 85.0 grams |
| 4 ounces | 113.4 grams |
| 8 ounces | 226.8 grams |
| 10 ounces | 283.5 grams |
| 12 ounces | 340.2 grams |
| 16 ounces | 453.6 grams |

# HERBAL SUPPLIERS

DANDELION BOTANICAL COMPANY   dandelionbotanical.com

FETTLE BOTANIC SUPPLY & COUNSEL   fettlebotanic.com

FOSTER FARM BOTANICALS   fosterfarmbotanicals.com

GAIA HERBS   gaiaherbs.com

MOUNTAIN ROSE HERBS   mountainroseherbs.com

OREGON'S WILD HARVEST   oregonswildharvest.com

PACIFIC BOTANICALS   pacificbotanicals.com

RADIANCE HERBS   radianceherbs.com

WISE WOMAN HERBALS   wisewomanherbals.com

WONDERLAND HERBS TEAS AND SPICES   360-733-0517 ·
wonderlandherbsteasspices.wordpress.com

# BOTANICAL NAMES of HERBS USED

AGRIMONY *Agrimonia eupatoria*

ALDER BUCKTHORN *Frangula alnus*

ALFALFA *Meticago sativa*

ANGELICA *Angelica archangelica*

ANISE *Pimpinella anisum*

ARNICA *Arnica montana*

ASAFOETIDA *Ferula assa-foetida*

ASHWAGANDHA *Withania somnifera*

BARBERRY *Berberis vulgaris*

BILBERRY *Vaccinium myrtillus*

BLACK COHOSH *Actaea racemosa* (also *Cimicifuga racemosa*)

BLACK WALNUT *Juglans nigra*

BLESSED THISTLE *Cnicus benedictus* (also *Centaurea benedicta*)

BONESET *Eupatorium perfoliatum*

BORAGE *Borago officinalis*

BUPLEURUM *Bupleurum chinense*

BURDOCK *Arctium lappa*

BUTCHER'S BROOM *Ruscus aculeatus*

CALENDULA *Calendula officinalis*

CALIFORNIA POPPY *Eschscholzia californica*

CARAWAY *Carum carvi*

CASCARA SAGRADA *Frangula purshiana*

CATNIP *Nepeta cataria*

CAT'S CLAW *Uncaria tomentosa*

CAYENNE *Capsicum annuum*

CEDAR *Thuja occidentalis*

CELANDINE *Chelidonium majus*

CELERY *Apium graveolens*

CENTAURY *Centaurium erythraea*

CHAMOMILE *Matricaria chamomilla*

CHAPARRAL *Larrea divaricata*

CHICKWEED *Stellaria media*

CLEAVERS *Galium aparine*

CLOVE *Syzygium aromaticum*

CLUB MOSS *Lycopodium clavatum*

COLTSFOOT *Tussilago farfara*

COMFREY *Symphytum officinale*

COUCH GRASS *Elymus repens*

CRAMP BARK *Viburnum opulus*

DAMIANA *Turnera diffusa*

DANDELION *Taraxacum officinale*

DEVIL'S CLUB *Oplopanax horridus*

DONG QUAI *Angelica sinensis*

ECHINACEA *Echinacea purpurea*

ELDER *Sambucus nigra*

ELECAMPANE *Inula helenium*

ELEUTHERO *Eleutherococcus senticosus*

EPIMEDIUM *Epimedium sagittatum*

EYEBRIGHT *Euphrasia officinalis*

FENNEL *Foeniculum vulgare*

FENUGREEK *Trigonella foenum-graecum*

FIGWORT *Scrophularia nodosa*

FO-TI *Polygonum multiflorum*

FRANKINCENSE *Boswellia serrata*

GENTIAN *Gentiana lutea*

GINGER *Zingiber officinale*

GINKGO *Ginkgo biloba*

GOAT'S RUE *Galega officinalis*

GOLDENSEAL *Hydrastis canadensis*

GOTU KOLA *Centella asiatica*

GRAND CACTUS *Selenicereus grandiflorus*

GRAVEL ROOT *Eupatorium purpureum*

GUARANA *Paullinia cupana*

HAWTHORN *Crataegus laevigata*

HIBISCUS *Hibiscus sabdariffa*

HOLY BASIL *Ocimum tenuiflorum*

HOPS *Humulus lupulus*

HOREHOUND *Marrubium vulgare*

HORSE CHESTNUT *Aesculus hippocastanum*

HORSERADISH *Armoracia rusticana*

HORSETAIL *Equisetum arvense*

HYDRANGEA *Hydrangea arborescens*

HYSSOP *Hyssopus officinalis*

JAMAICAN DOGWOOD *Piscidia piscipula*

JUNIPER *Juniperus communis*

KAVA KAVA *Piper methysticum*

LADY'S MANTLE *Alchemilla vulgaris*

LAVENDER *Lavendula* species

LEMON BALM *Melissa officinalis*

LEMONGRASS *Cymbopogon* species

LICORICE *Glycyrrhiza glabra*

LINDEN  *Tilia americana*

LION'S MANE  *Hericium erinaceus*

LOBELIA  *lobelia inflata*

LOMATIUM  *Lomatium dissectum*

MACA  *Lepidium meyenii*

MAITAKE  *Grifola frondosa*

MARSHMALLOW  *Althaea officinalis*

MEADOWSWEET  *Filipendula ulmaria*

MILK THISTLE  *Silybum marianum*

MOTHERWORT  *Leonurus cardiaca*

MUGWORT  *Artemisia vulgaris*

MULLEIN  *Verbascum thapsus*

MYRRH  *Commiphora myrrha*

NETTLE  *Urtica dioica*

OATSTRAW  *Avena sativa*

OREGON GRAPE  *Mahonia aquifolium*

OSHA  *Ligusticum porteri*

PARTRIDGE BERRY  *Mitchella repens*

PASSIONFLOWER  *Passiflora incarnata*

PAU D'ARCO  *Tabebuia avellanedae*

PEPPERMINT  *Mentha ×piperita*

PINE  *Pinus pinaster*

PIPSISSEWA  *Chimaphila umbellata*

PLANTAIN  *Plantago major*

PLEURISY ROOT  *Asclepias tuberosa*

POKE  *Phytolaca americana*

POPLAR  *Populus tremuloides*

PRICKLY ASH  *Zanthoxylum clava-herculis*

RASPBERRY  *Rubus idaeus*

RED CLOVER  *Trifolium pratense*

RED ROOT  *Amaranthus retroflexus*

REISHI  *Ganoderma applanatum* (also *G. lucidum, G. oregonense, G. tsugae*)

RHODIOLA  *Rhodiola rosea*

ROOIBOS  *Aspalanthus linearis*

ROSE  *Rosa* species

ROSEMARY  *Rosmarinus officinalis*

SAFFLOWER  *Carthamus tinctorius*

SAGE  *Salvia officinalis*

SAW PALMETTO  *Serenoa repens*

SCHISANDRA  *Schisandra chinensis*

SHATAVARI  *Asparagus racemosus*

SHEPHERD'S PURSE  *Capsella bursa-pastoris*

SHIITAKE  *Lentinula edodes*

SILK TASSEL  *Garrya elliptica*

SKULLCAP  *Scutellaria lateriflora*

SLIPPERY ELM  *Ulmus rubra*

SPEARMINT  *Mentha spicata*

SPILANTHES  *Spilanthes acmella*

ST. JOHN'S WORT  *Hypericum perforatum*

STONE ROOT  *Collinsonia canadensis*

SUMAC  *Rhus glabra*

THYME  *Thymus vulgaris*

TRIBULUS  *Tribulus terrestris*

TURKEY RHUBARB  *Rheum palmatum*

TURMERIC  *Curcuma longa*

USNEA  *Usnea barbata*

VALERIAN  *Valeriana officinalis*

VERVAIN  *Verbena officinalis*

VIOLET  *Viola odorata*

VITEX  *Vitex agnus-castus*

WHITE OAK  *Quercus alba*

WHITE WILLOW  *Salix alba*

WILD CHERRY  *Prunus serotina*

WILD LETTUCE  *Lactuca virosa*

WILD YAM  *Dioscorea villosa*

WIREWEED  *Sida acuta*

WOOD BETTONY  *Stachys officinalis*

WORMWOOD  *Artemisia absinthium*

YARROW  *Achillea millefolium*

YELLOW DOCK  *Rumex crispus*

YERBA SANTA  *Eriodictyon californicum*

YOHIMBE  *Pausinystalia johimbe*

YUCCA  *Yucca glauca*

# FURTHER READING

Buhner, Stephen Harrod. 2012. *Herbal Antibiotics*, 2nd ed. North Adams, MA: Storey.

Crow, Tis Mal. 2001. *Native Plants, Native Healing: Traditional Muskogee Way.* Summertown, TN: Native Voices.

Deitsch, Irene. 2016. *Tussie-Mussies: A Collector's Guide to Victorian Posy Holders.* Palo Alto, CA: Irene Deitsch.

Duke, James A. 2000. *The Green Pharmacy Herbal Handbook.* Emmaus, PA: Rodale.

Gladstar, Rosemary. 2012. *Rosemary Gladstar's Medicinal Herbs: A Beginner's Guide*, 9th ed. North Adams, MA: Storey.

Green, James. 2007. *The Male Herbal: The Definitive Health Care Book for Men and Boys*, 2nd ed. Berkeley, CA: Crossing Press.

Hoffmann, David. 1989. *The Herbal Handbook: A User's Guide to Medical Herbalism.* Rochester, VT: Inner Traditions.

———. 1993. *An Elders' Herbal: Natural Techniques for Health and Vitality.* Rochester, VT: Healing Arts Press.

Kloos, Scott. 2017. *Pacific Northwest Medicinal Plants.* Portland, OR: Timber Press.

Kloss, Jethro. 1939. *Back to Eden*. Loma Linda, CA: Back to Eden Books.

Laufer, Geraldine Adamich. 2000. *Tussie-Mussies: The Language of Flowers*. New York, NY: Workman.

Light, Phyllis D. 2018. *Southern Folk Medicine: Healing Traditions from the Appalachian Fields and Forests*. Berkeley, CA: North Atlantic Books.

Pursell, JJ. 2015. *The Herbal Apothecary: 100 Medicinal Herbs and How to Use Them*. Portland, OR: Timber Press.

– 2018. The Woman's Herbal Apothecary: 200 Natural Remedies for Healing, Hormone Balance, Beauty and Longevity, and Creating Calm. Beverly, MA: Fair Winds Press.

Stuart, Malcolm, ed. 1979. *The Encyclopedia of Herbs and Herbalism*. New York, NY: Grosset and Dunlap.

# ACKNOWLEDGMENTS

When I get to this point I always take a moment and reflect back on the process of manifesting the book you hold in your hands. I am flooded with faces, memories, and environments that were all part of its creation. First I must thank my family: my husband, Brian, who watched the kids endless weekends so I could reach my goal; my kids, who never held it against me when I went off to sit countless hours in the library or Peet's coffeehouse; my mom, who stepped in often to support; and my sister, brother-in-law, and nieces, who knew when to connect and offer some fun downtime with the family. This book was written over a summer—thank goodness for family pool time!

Stacee Lawrence, editor extraordinaire at Timber, made everything so easy and pleasant that it barely felt like work. I truly felt supported by her and knew that she always had my back. Thank you, Stacee! And of course, Shawn Linehan—my sister friend. You've ruined it for all other photographers because your perfection through the lens is now something I cannot live without. Thank you for your patience, wise counsel, and making my book beautiful. The Timber design team—Patrick, Sarah, and Hillary—made me feel more supported than I ever have before at a photo shoot. Thank you for getting intimate with me, holding the space, and bringing the vision to life on the pages of this book. You are all so amazing! And last—Ms. Lorraine. Oh my goodness! Without your never-ending patience and the delicate and incredibly fine editing job you've done with this book, it wouldn't be half of what it is. No one really understands how much editors do—but they really do sprinkle the magic that pulls it all together. Thank you, Lorraine—it has been a pleasure!

As always, I end with giving thanks to all of the teachers, herbalists, and plant doctors, and to the plants themselves, for giving me a chance and showing me the way into your world. It has been an honor and a privilege to share time and space with you.

Kind regards,
JJ

# PHOTO CREDITS

All photos, excepting those noted below, courtesy of Shawn Linehan.

Leoadec, page 64

LuckyStarr, page 66

Qwert1234, page 64

Reaperman, page 59

Schnobby, page 69

Teun Spaans, page 64

Forest & Kim Starr, page 75

James Steakley, page 65

Ramon FVelasquez, page 68

H. Zell, pages 68, 70

Roland zh, page 60

*Used under the Creative Commons*
  *Attribution-Share Alike 4.0*
  *International license*
Bff, page 75

R. A. Nonenmacher, page 70

Salix, page 74

Vinayaraj, page 58

*Used under the GNU Free*
  *Documentation license*
Liné1, page 73

Loadmaster (David R. Tribble), page 73

# INDEX

283

286

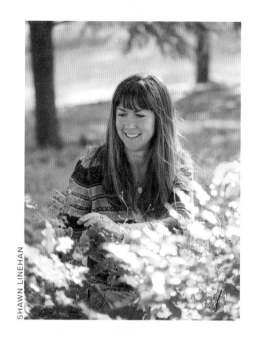

DR. JJ PURSELL is a board-certified naturopathic physician and licensed acupuncturist and has worked with medicinal herbs for more than twenty years. Having spent many hours on her father's flower farm, she learned to love plants at an early age. She began working at herb farms and herb shops, which inspired her to enroll in graduate studies in health and medicine. While in school, having returned to the urban life, she missed the plants and the community that an herb shop offers. She opened The Herb Shoppe, now Fettle Botanic Supply & Counsel (fettlebotanic.com), while finishing her degree in Portland, Oregon. She has taught and trained with herbalists all over the world but prefers the practice of close-to-home–grown Western herbs.

Fettle focuses on offering the most vital organic herbs available, while sustaining local growers. Over the years, Fettle has received countless words of thanks for all it has to offer and has been asked by many patrons to open shops in other parts of the country. With the continued success of both businesses, Fettle is seeking partners who are passionate about community and herbal medicine and would like to own a Fettle shop in their city.

Fettle was voted "the best apothecary in Portland" by *Willamette Week* and was written up in *Portland Monthly* magazine and *The L Magazine* in New York City. JJ and her shop have been featured in several blogs and Tumblr sites, including Gardenista, White & Warren Inspired, Kale and Coriander, Portland Healing Project, PoppySwap, and Girl Gift Gather. JJ appeared on "Green Living," a BCAT television show in Brooklyn; the "Bread and Roses" radio show on Portland's KBOO; and "Wise Woman Radio" with Susun Weed. She is the author of *The Herbal Apothecary: 100 Medicinal Herbs and How to Use Them*, from Timber Press. She is also included in the book *Curing Canine Cancer*. She has her own YouTube channel for those who want to learn more about making herbal medicine.